M. EBADI, Ph.D.

International Review of

EXPERIMENTAL PATHOLOGY

Volume 34

CYTOKINE-INDUCED PATHOLOGY
PART B: Inflammatory Cytokines, Receptors, and Disease

International Review of
EXPERIMENTAL PATHOLOGY

Volume 34
CYTOKINE-INDUCED PATHOLOGY
PART B: Inflammatory Cytokines, Receptors, and Disease

Edited by

G. W. Richter
Department of Pathology
University of Rochester Medical Center
Rochester, New York

Kim Solez
Department of Pathology
Faculty of Medicine
University of Alberta
Edmonton, Alberta
Canada

Guest Editor

Bernhard Ryffel
Institut für Toxikologie
Eidgenössischen Technischen Hochschule
Universität Zürich
Schwerzenbach/Zürich
Switzerland

ACADEMIC PRESS, INC.
Harcourt Brace Jovanovich, Publishers
San Diego   New York   Boston   London   Sydney   Tokyo   Toronto

Contents

Section I
PATHOLOGY INDUCED BY INFLAMMATORY CYTOKINES

Introduction

Pathophysiologic Alterations Induced by Tumor Necrosis Factor

Daniel G. Remick and Steven L. Kunkel

In Vitro and *in Vivo* Activity and Pathophysiology of Human Interleukin-8 and Related Peptides

Roland Zwahlen, Alfred Walz, and Antal Rot

Pathology of Recombinant Human Transforming Growth Factor-β1 in Rats and Rabbits

Timothy G. Terrell, Peter K. Working, C. Paul Chow, and James D. Green

Pathology Induced by Leukemia Inhibitory Factor

Bernhard Ryffel

Comparative Pathology of Recombinant Murine Interferon-γ in Mice and Recombinant Human Interferon-γ in Cynomolgus Monkeys

Timothy G. Terrell and James D. Green

Section II
CYTOKINE RECEPTORS

Introduction to Cytokine Receptors: Structure and Signal Transduction

Pharmacokinetic Parameters and Biodistribution of Soluble Cytokine Receptors

Cindy A. Jacobs, M. Patricia Beckmann, Ken Mohler, Charles R. Maliszewski, William C. Fanslow, and David H. Lynch

Immunomodulation with Soluble IFN-γ Receptor: Preliminary Study

Laurence Ozmen, Michael Fountoulakis, Reiner Gentz, and Gianni Garotta

TNF Receptor Distribution in Human Tissues

Bernhard Ryffel and M. J. Mihatsch

Section III
ROLE OF CYTOKINES IN DISEASE

Tumor Necrosis Factor/Cachectin as an Effector of T Cell-Dependent Immunopathology

Georges E. Grau, Paul-Henri Lambert, Pierre Vassalli, and Pierre-François Piguet

Cytokines Involved in Pulmonary Fibrosis

Pierre-François Piguet

Immune-Mediated Injury in Bacterial Meningitis

Karl Frei, Daniela Piani, Hans-Walter Pfister, and Adriano Fontana

Contributors

Numbers in parentheses indicate the pages on which the authors' contributions begin.

Kathy Barrett, Sunley Research Institute, London, England (105).

M. Patricia Beckmann, Immunex Corporation, Seattle, Washington 98101 (123).

C. Paul Chow, Department of Safety Evaluation, Genentech, Inc., South San Francisco, California 94080 (43).

William C. Fanslow, Immunex Corporation, Seattle, Washington 98101 (123).

Adriano Fontana, Section of Clinical Immunology, Department of Neurosurgery, University Hospital, CH-8044 Zürich, Switzerland (183).

Michael Fountoulakis, Pharmaceutical Research, New Technologies, Hoffmann-La Roche Ltd., CH-4002 Basel, Switzerland (137).

Brian Foxwell, Sunley Research Institute, London, England (105).

Karl Frei, Section of Clinical Immunology, Department of Neurosurgery, University Hospital, CH-8044 Zürich, Switzerland (183).

Gianni Garotta, Pharmaceutical Research, New Technologies, Hoffman-La Roche Ltd., Ch-4002 Basel, Switzerland (137).

Reiner Gentz, Pharmaceutical Research, New Technologies, Hoffman-La Roche Ltd., Ch-4002 Basel, Switzerland (137).

Georges E. Grau, Department of Pathology, WHO-IRTC, University of Geneva, CH-1211 Geneva 4, Switzerland (159).

James D. Green, Department of Safety Evaluation, Genentech, Inc., South San Francisco, California 94080 (43,73).

Cindy A. Jacobs, Immunex Corporation, Seattle, Washington 98101 (123).

Thomas C. Jones, Clinical Research, Sandoz Pharma Ltd., CH-4002 Basel, Switzerland (209).

Steven L. Kunkel, Department of Pathology, University of Michigan Medical School, Ann Arbor, Michigan 48109 (7).

Paul-Henri Lambert, Department of Pathology, WHO-IRTC, University of Geneva, CH-1211 Geneva 4, Switzerland (159).

Gerhard Leitz, Corporate Medicine, Boehringer Ingelheim, Ingelheim, Germany (193).

David H. Lynch, Immunex Corporation, Seattle, Washington 98101 (123).

Charles R. Maliszewski, Immunex Corporation, Seattle, Washington 98101 (123).

M. J. Mihatsch, Institut für Pathologie, Universität Basel, CH-4003 Basel, Switzerland (149).

Ken Mohler, Immunex Corporation, Seattle, Washington 98101 (123).

Laurence Ozmen, Pharmaceutical Research, New Technologies, Hoffman-La Roche Ltd., CH-4002 Basel, Switzerland (137).

Hans-Walter Pfister, Department of Neurology, University of Munich, Munich, Germany (183).

Daniela Piani, Section of Clinical Immunology, Department of Neurosurgery, University Hospital, CH-8044 Zürich, Switzerland (183).

Pierre-François Piguet, Départment de Pathologie, Université de Genève, CH-1211 Genève 4, Switzerland (159,173).

Daniel G. Remick, Department of Pathology, University of Michigan Medical School, Ann Arbor, Michigan 48109 (7).

Frank Rosenkaimer, Corporate Medicine, Boehringer Ingelheim, Ingelheim, Germany (193).

Antal Rot, Sandoz Forschungsinstitut, A-1235 Vienna, Austria (27).

Bernhard Ryffel, Institut für Toxikologie, Eidgenössischen Technischen Hochschule, Universität Zürich, CH-8603 Schwerzenbach/Zürich, Switzerland (3,69,149).

Gerhard G. Steinmann, Clinical Research, Boehringer Ingelheim, D-7950 Biberach, Germany (193).

Angelika C. Stern, Clinical Research, Sandoz Pharma Ltd., CH-4002 Basel, Switzerland (209).

Timothy G. Terrell, Department of Safety Evaluation, Genentech, Inc., South San Francisco, California 94080 (43,73).

Pierre Vassalli, Department of Pathology, WHO-IRTC, University of Geneva, CH-1211 Geneva 4, Switzerland (159).

Alfred Walz, Theodor Kocher Institut, Universität Bern, CH-3001 Bern 9, Switzerland (27).

Peter K. Working, Department of Pharmacology and Toxicology, Liposome Technologies, Inc., Menlo Park, California 94025 (43).

Roland Zwahlen, Institut für Tierpathologie, Universität Bern, CH-3001 Bern 9, Switzerland (27).

Preface

Cytokines and growth factors play an important regulatory role in the cross talk of different cell systems. Cytokines are regulatory peptides that are produced by many different cell types in the body, and often have pleiotropic regulatory effects on hemopoietic, lymphoid, and inflammatory cells. Recent developments in molecular biology have allowed the cloning and production of a variety of recombinant growth factors. With the availability of pure recombinant proteins, neutralizing antibody, and the rapid development of biological models, it became possible to define the physiological roles of many of these growth factors. Furthermore, the clinical use of hemopoietic growth factors such as erythropoietin, granulocyte, and granulocyte–monocyte colony stimulating factors has recently been introduced in different disease conditions.

Although these growth factors and cytokines are normally produced by the body, the exogenous and systemic administration of high doses of these growth factors may cause pathology.

For these volumes, I have asked experts in pathology to present experimental findings obtained from the most recently studied cytokines and growth factors. I am very pleased that most of the contributions include novel and, to a large extent, unpublished experimental findings, which might help us to understand the physiological and pathological changes associated with these peptides. I appreciate very much the efforts of many scientists from around the world who have contributed to this volume, and I am convinced that it represents a unique review on cytokine pathology.

These volumes are essentially based on a workshop held in Basel, Switzerland (August, 1991), which was organized together with my colleagues T. Hayes, M. J. Mihatsch, and G. Zbinden. The realization of the workshop was only made possible by generous financial support from the Sandoz Pharma Corporation in Basel.

Bernhard Ryffel

Section I

PATHOLOGY INDUCED BY INFLAMMATORY CYTOKINES

Introduction

Bernhard Ryffel
Institut für Toxikologie
Eidgenössischen Technischen Hochschule
Universität Zürich
CH-8603 Schwerzenbach/Zürich, Switzerland

Tissue injury or exposure of an organism to pathogenic stimuli triggers a number of host cellular defense mechanisms, leading to inflammation. Locally released mediators from endothelial cells, macrophages, mast cells, and connective tissue cells mediate the early inflammatory reaction. These early mediators include bradykinin and histamine (which are potent vasodilators), complement components, prostaglandins, kinins, platelet-activating factor, and a number of granulocyte-derived proteases. Only recently has the role of the cytokines in the recruitment of cells at the site of inflammation, in activation of immunoeffector cells, including the phagocytic system, and in tissue repair been recognized (see Table I).

In this work the biological effects of interferon-γ, tumor necrosis factor, interleukin-8, transforming growth factor-β, and leukemia inhibitory factor are described in experimental animals. It is obvious that the biological activity of this group of cytokines is not limited to inflammatory processes, because inflammation, immune response, and to some extent hematopoiesis are tightly linked. Thus, the segregation of cytokines into functional groups is arbitrary and may only indicate the main biological activity of the molecule. Thus, the pleiotropic cytokines IL-1 and IL-6 play an important role in inflammatory reactions.

I. INTERFERON-γ

Interferon-γ (IFN-γ; also known as immune interferon) is mainly produced by activated T lymphocytes and possibly by natural killer cells. Other members of the interferon family include fibroblast-derived interferon-α and leukocyte-derived interferon-β.

Cloned human IFN-γ encodes a mature protein of 143 amino acids. Active IFN-γ is a homodimeric molecule with a molecular mass of 45 kDa. Murine IFN-γ has only 45% homology to the human molecule at the protein level. The difference in structure is large enough that there is no cross-reactivity of the biological effects of human and mouse IFN-γ. In contrast, the homology

Table I. Molecular Characteristics of Human Inflammatory Cytokines

Cytokine	Molecular mass (kDa)		Homology with mouse protein (%)	Source	Activity	Receptor
Interferon-γ	45	(dimer)	45	T lymphocytes	Virus, macrophages, granulocytes, lymphocytes	p80
TNF-α	45	(trimer)	80	Macophages	Lymphocytes, epithelium	p55/p75
TNF-β	60	(trimer)	75	T lymphocytes	Endothelium, tumor cells	p55/p75
IL-8	8		80	Lymphocytes, macrophages	Chemotaxis	p90

of mouse and rat IFN-γ is high, and thus the two molecules are interchangeable for the two species.

All interferons have antiviral activity; interferon-γ has, in addition, regulatory functions for macrophages (macrophage activation), T and B lymphocytes, and granulocytes. Among interferons, interferon-γ is the most effective inducer of *de novo* synthesis of major histocompatibility (MHC) class II antigens in macrophages in addition to stimulation of class I antigens. Interferon-γ synergizes with lipopolysaccharide (LPS)-induced production of IL-1, IL-6, and tumor necrosis factor-α (TNF-α) in macrophages. Besides the macrophage activation, interferon-γ has effects on T and B lymphocytes. In T lymphocytes interferon-γ possibly acts as an autocrine or paracrine growth factor.

Interferon-γ receptors are widely distributed in tissues and have been recently cloned. The homology of the human and murine receptor proteins are low and no cross-reactivity occurs with the ligands. The biological effect *in vivo,* especially in infectious diseases and malignancies, has been evaluated and exploited in specific clinical situations.

II. TUMOR NECROSIS FACTOR

An investigation of the antitumor effect of the LPS component of endotoxin derived from gram-negative bacteria led to the discovery of the TNF molecule, which has direct tumoricidal activity against a range of tumor cells *in vitro.* Activated macrophages are the main cellular source of TNF-α. A second type of TNF molecule, isolated from activated T lymphocytes, is called lymphotoxin, or TNF-β. Both TNF molecules have been molecularly defined and consist of three identical monomeric subunits, 17 kDa each for TNF-α and 20 kDA each for TNF-β.

The homology between TNF-α and -β is only 36% at the amino acid level. From an evolutionary point of view, the two molecules are probably derived from a common ancestral gene. The mouse homologues of TNF-α and -β are also only distantly related. The homology between mouse and human TNF-α, however, is about 80% at the amino acid level and TNF-β shows approximately 75% overall homology for the two species. Based on these considerations, a partial cross-reactivity of human TNF-α and -β for biological activity on murine cells is predictable.

Both TNF molecules bind to widely distributed receptors in tissues. Despite the marked difference in amino sequences, TNF-α and TNF-β bind to common cell surface receptors. The human TNF receptor is composed of a 55- and a 75-kDa protein. Both receptor proteins bind the TNF molecules independently and the possibility that the two receptor proteins mediate a different biological effect is presently under investigation.

The biological activities of TNF-α and -β are quite similar and are characterized by a broad spectrum of action, including activation of T and B lymphocytes, activation of macrophages and granulocytes, inhibition of hematopoiesis, a cytotoxic effect for tumor cells, and activation of endothelial cells. Furthermore, these molecules cause cachexia after *in vivo* administration. The tumoricidal properties of TNF molecules are presently being tested in cancer patients.

III. INTERLEUKIN-8

IL-8 belongs to a large family of low-molecular-weight peptides with chemotactic activity for neutrophilic granulocytes. (See Zwahlen *et al.,* this volume, for a discussion of the molecular characteristics and biological properties of IL-8.) In contrast to other activators of neutrophilic granulocytes, such as GM-CSF, local injection of IL-8 causes an accumulation of granulocytes, but does not cause activation of these cells or tissue destruction.

References

Aguet, M., Dembic, C., and Merlin, G. (1988). *Cell* **55,** 273.
Beutler, B., Greenwald, D., and Hulmes, J. D. (1985). *Nature (London)* **316,** 552.
Gray, P. W., and Goeddel, D. V. (1982). *Nature (London)* **298,** 859.
Gray, P. W., and Goeddel, D. V. (1983). *Proc. Nat. Acad. Sci. U.S.A.* **80,** 5842.
Gray, P. W., Aggarwal, B. B., Benton, C. V., *et al.* (1984). *Nature (London)* **312,** 721.
Hacklett, R. J., Davis, L. S., and Lipsky, P. E. (1988). *J. Immunol.* **140,** 2639.
Jones, E. Y., Stuart, D. I., and Walker, N. P. C. (1989). *Nature (London)* **338,** 225.

Larsen, C. G., Anderson, A. O., Appella, E., *et al.* (1988). *Science* **243,** 1464.
Matsushima, K., Morishita, K., Yoshimura, T., *et al.* (1988). *J. Exp. Med.* **167,** 1883.
Nathan, C. F. (1987). *J. Clin. Invest.* **79,** 319.
Pennica, D., Newin, G. E., Hayflick, J. S., *et al.* (1984). *Nature (London)* **312,** 724.
Samanta, A. K., Oppenheim, J. J., and Matsuhima, K. (1989). *J. Exptl. Med.* **169,** 1185.

Pathophysiologic Alterations Induced by Tumor Necrosis Factor

Daniel G. Remick and Steven L. Kunkel
Department of Pathology
University of Michigan Medical School
Ann Arbor, Michigan 48109

I. INTRODUCTION

Tumor necrosis factor-α (TNF) is a small peptide mediator secreted primarily by cells of monocyte lineage. This 17,000-Da cytokine exerts multiple effects both *in vitro* and *in vivo*. TNF was first described as an oncolytic agent directed against solid tumors (Carswell *et al.,* 1975), but further work began to disclose its broad range of activity. TNF has been implicated in the pathogenesis of several diseases and inflammatory conditions, including rejection of transplanted solid organs (Maury and Teppo, 1987), congestive heart failure (Levine *et al.,* 1990), arthritis (Saxne *et al.,* 1988), parasitic infections (Scuderi *et al.,* 1986), glomerulonephritis (Remick, 1991), and acquired immunodeficiency syndrome (Lahdevirta *et al.,* 1988). It must be mentioned that this is by no means a complete list of diseases in which TNF has been implicated in the altered pathophysiology.

The strongest evidence for TNF participation in a disease state is found in the data describing TNF and septic shock. Data supporting the hypothesis that TNF mediates septic shock have been provided by multiple independent laboratories and consist of four parts. First, in experimental animal models of septic shock, TNF is produced and secreted into the circulation within 1 to 2 hr. The rapid production of TNF is observed in humans (Michie *et al.,* 1988), rabbits (Beutler *et al.,* 1985b; Mathison *et al.,* 1988), and rodents (Waage, 1987; Remick *et al.,* 1989). The second line of evidence for the role of TNF is the detection of TNF in the serum of patients in septic shock (Waage *et al.,* 1987). In this now classic study, TNF was present in the serum of 10 of 11 patients who died, but was in the serum of only 6 of 68 survivors. All patients with greater than 100 pg/ml of TNF in their serum died. More recent work has confirmed this earlier report (Debets *et al.,* 1989; Marks *et al.,* 1990). The third piece of information is given by experiments wherein antibodies to TNF will prevent the lethality observed after injection of endotoxin (Beutler *et al.,* 1985a) or live gram-negative bacteria (Tracey *et al.,* 1987a). The study with live bacteria raised some concerns about potential endotoxin contamination in the antibody preparation, because the antibody needed to be given 2 hr prior to the bacteria in order to be efficacious. Work by Chong and Huston (1987) had demonstrated that endotoxin contamination in antibody preparations could confer nonspecific protection if the antibodies were given 2 hr prior to lipopolysaccharide (LPS). These doubts were alleviated by Hinshaw *et al.* (1990), who started the antibody treatment after 30 min of infusion of bacteria, and were still able to confer protection. The last piece of evidence for the role of TNF became available when sufficient amounts of recombinant material could be provided to investigators. Workers in several labs have been able to inject this purified material into experimental animals and induce altered pathophysiology and organ injury. Tracy *et al.* (1986) first reported that injection of recombinant human TNF (rHuTNF) would induce shock and tissue injury. Since that initial report, we and other groups have provided additional evidence of the effects of TNF injection into experimental animals. These data represent the focus of this review.

II. TNF-INDUCED PERIPHERAL BLOOD ALTERATIONS

A. Neutrophilia and Lymphopenia

Injection of rHuTNF into mice results in the rapid induction of lymphopenia and neutrophilia (Remick *et al.,* 1986). For our experiments, we used purified, recombinant human TNF, which was the generous gift of Cetus Corporation (Emeryville, California). The kinetics of these peripheral blood alterations are extremely rapid, with statistically significant alterations occurring within 1 hr. The lymphopenia and neutrophilia are both absolute and relative; that is, there is both a decrease in the percentage of lymphocytes as well as a decrease in the total number of circulating lymphocytes. Because the number of neutrophils is increasing while the lymphocytes are decreasing, in our experiments the total white count never changes. The peripheral blood alterations are the parameters most sensitive to change after injection of rHuTNF, with significant relative lymphopenia and neutrophilia documented with as little as 10 ng/mouse (0.45 μg/kg body weight; Remick *et al.,* 1987). Whereas the relative changes were quite reproducible, the absolute changes did not occur until reaching a dose of 1000 ng/mouse for the lymphopenia and 100 ng/mouse for the neutrophilia. These peripheral blood changes persisted for at least 6 hr, which was the end of the experiment. At the 6-hr time point there was the beginning of a return to normal values. Since our original observation, similar peripheral blood alterations after injection of rHuTNF have been reported by Ulich *et al.* (1987, 1989).

B. Mechanisms of Peripheral Blood Changes

There are multiple methods whereby the neutrophilia and lymphopenia may occur. The neutrophilia may be due to recruitment of new cells from the bone marrow, or demargination of cells from blood vessel walls. In fact, the neutrophilia is due to a combination of both mechanisms. We (Remick *et al.,* 1986) examined peripheral blood smears to look for the presence of immature neutrophils, as well as mature neutrophils. Both the mature and immature forms of neutrophils were present. Ulich *et al.* (1987) performed differentials from the bone marrow of rats treated with rHuTNF and found a decrease in the number of band and segmented myeloid forms, providing additional evidence that TNF induces recruitment of neutrophils from the bone marrow. This laboratory also evaluated the role that endogenous release of other cytokines may play, and showed that in rats the second wave of neutrophilia is most likely due to endogenous release of interleukin-1 (Ulich *et al.,* 1989).

The mechanism of lymphopenia may also be multifactorial. TNF has been shown to up-regulate adhesion molecules on endothelial cells, which could then bind the lymphocytes. TNF could also be directly toxic to lymphocytes, inducing damage such that they are then cleared by the reticuloendothelial system. Playfair *et al.* (1982) reported that serum that contained tumor-necrotizing capacity (i.e., probably contained TNF) was toxic to murine B cells. We performed flow-cytometric phenotyping to determine if there was specific loss of a subset of lymphocytes after injection of rHuTNF. Although B cells were decreased more than T cells or natural killer cells, this reduction could not account for the entire reduction in lymphocytes (Remick *et al.,* 1987). We also evaluated the *in vitro* toxicity of TNF toward normal lymphocytes. Even in the presence of complement, there was no direct toxicity (Kunkel *et al.,* 1989). Ulich also sought to determine if there was reduced recirculation of lymphocytes in the thoracic duct after injection of rHuTNF in rats and found no decrease. These experiments ruled out the possibility that the reduction in circulating lymphocytes was due to failure of the cells to be returned to the peripheral blood (Ulich *et al.,* 1989).

C. Controls for Endotoxin Contamination

It is critical to control for the presence of endotoxin in the recombinant cytokine preparations, for several reasons. One of the central hypotheses is that during many *in vivo* inflammatory conditions a challenge induces the production of cytokines, which then cause the tissue damage. However, if the recombinant preparation contains significant endotoxin, then an investigator may be inadvertently studying the effects of endotoxin and not the cytokine. This is especially important with recombinant materials, because most of them were produced in the gram-negative bacteria *Escherichia coli.* To ensure that our data concerning the peripheral blood changes were due to TNF and not contaminating endotoxin, we performed extensive controls. As shown in Fig. 1, these multiple controls rule out possible endotoxin contamination (Remick *et al.,* 1986). Injection of 1 μg of TNF resulted in the rapid induction of the lymphopenia and neutrophilia, compared to normal saline controls. TNF is rapidly inactivated by heating to 95°C for 15 min whereas endotoxin is remarkably resistant to heating. Heat inactivation of the TNF preparation completely abolished its ability to induce peripheral blood alterations. Although endotoxin was not detectable in the rHuTNF preparation, it was possible that levels below the detection limits of the assay were present. We therefore injected 1 ng of lipopolysaccharide, the amount of LPS that could theoretically be present in 1 μg of TNF. This amount of LPS did not induce changes. Finally, polymyxin B will bind to and inactivate LPS (Neter *et al.,* 1958), but addition of polymyxin B to the TNF did not block its activity.

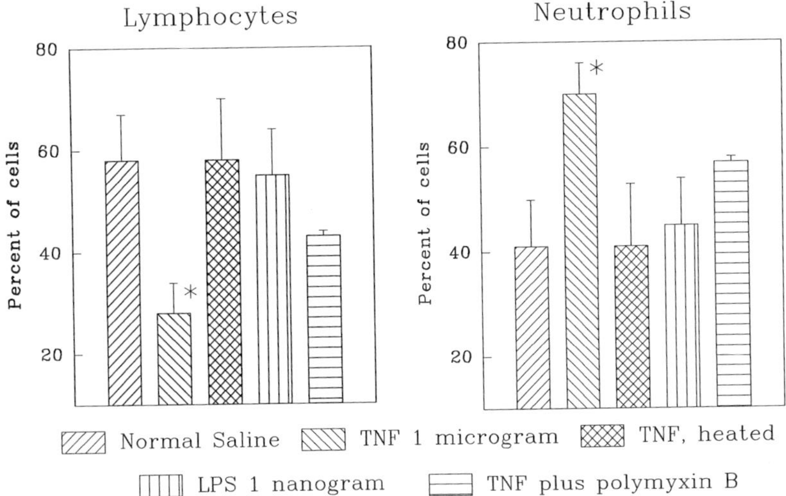

Fig. 1. Controls for endotoxin contamination in rHuTNF preparation. rHuTNF (1 μg) was injected intravenously in a 200-μl volume, and the peripheral blood was evaluated 2 hr later. TNF induced neutrophilia and lymphopenia; heat inactivation prevented these changes. LPS at the maximum contaminating dose did alter the peripheral blood constituents, and mixing the TNF with polymyxin B did not block changes. Each value is the mean $\pm$ SD for three to eight mice. *, $p < 0.05$ compared to the normal saline control.

An additional control was done using C3H/H3J mice. These mice have a defective LPS-response gene (Watson *et al.,* 1978) and are thus not sensitive to the effects of endotoxin. Figure 2 shows a flow-cytometric evaluation of the peripheral blood 2 hr after injection of 1 μg of rHuTNF. These mice also developed a neutrophilia and lymphopenia, providing further evidence that the changes were not due to endotoxin contamination.

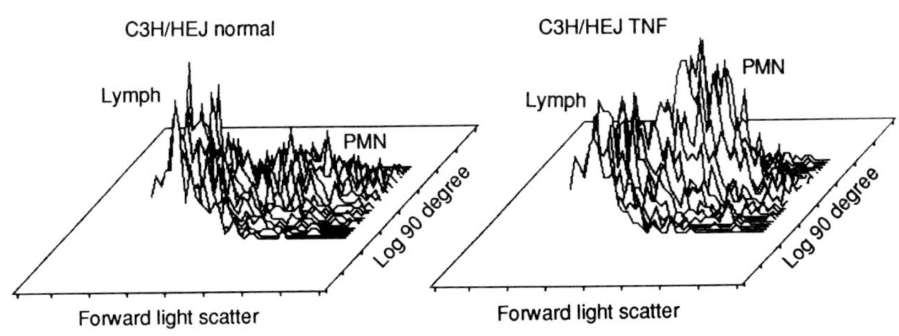

Fig. 2. Flow cytometric study of peripheral blood. C3H/HeJ mice were injected with 1 μg/mouse of rHuTNF and the peripheral blood was evaluated 2 hr later. Lymphocytes and neutrophils were identified by their light-scatter characteristics. rHuTNF induced lymphopenia and neutrophilia compared to the control mice, which were injected with vehicle alone.

III. ORGAN INJURY INDUCED BY TNF

Injection of purified, recombinant TNF to experimental animals, or to cancer patients (Spriggs *et al.,* 1988) as a form of therapy, can result in severe, widespread organ injury. Though injection of TNF can be used to study the toxicity of oncolytic agents, many investigators are using recombinant TNF in an attempt to mimic the pathophysiologic alterations that are observed in septic shock. During bacterial sepsis, or after injection of LPS, a shocklike state often ensues. The animals develop fever malaise and hypotension; these changes are believed to be due to the endogenous release of TNF by the cells of the reticuloendothelial system.

A. Gross Observations

We began our investigations into the tissue injury in 1986, using purified, recombinant human TNF. The experimental approach was very simple. Increasing doses of TNF were injected intravenously and the animals were observed until sacrifice. Adult female CBA/J mice were used throughout the study (Remick *et al.,* 1987). After sacrifice, complete gross and microscopic examinations were performed. As described above, the most sensitive parameter for detecting an effect of TNF was the alteration in peripheral blood constituents. At higher doses, above 1μg/mouse ($45\ \mu$g/kg body weight), it was clear that this inflammatory peptide was toxic. Prior to sacrifice, the animals became lethargic and huddled together in a corner of the cage. Ruffled fur, particularly on the upper portion of the back, provided evidence of piloerection. Diarrhea also developed, and at doses above $1\ \mu$g/mouse all of the mice developed loose stools. These effects developed rapidly, with the mice becoming visibly ill within 1 hr. We focused our work on the 2hr time point after intravenous injection of rHuTNF, because the toxicology was well developed by this time and we had previously documented the peripheral blood alterations.

Upon opening the abdomen at the time of sacrifice, it was immediately apparent that there was severe intestinal injury. The majority of the small intestine was dilated and filled with edema fluid and loose, liquid stool. The large intestine was much less affected, although there were some focal areas of slight dilatation. In our initial experiments, 25% of the animals treated with 10μg/mouse of rHuTNF had intussusception of the ileocecal valve into the cecum. The remainder of the organs appeared grossly normal.

B. Microscopic Alterations

Microscopic examination was performed on tissues to confirm the gross impressions that the intestines were primarily affected. The doses that were used in these studies ranged from 0.001 to 10 μg. Organ injury was observed only at the 1- and 10-μg doses.

Routine microscopy was done on heart, lung, liver, kidney, spleen, and intestines. We took great care to gently flush the lumen of the intestines with formalin to ensure prompt fixation, because preliminary experiments showed some mild autolysis of the intestinal mucosa in controls. Adherence to a careful protocol permitted us to discern the toxic effects of TNF. It should be noted that we could find no evidence of damage in any organs other than the intestines. However, we did not examine the uterus, which has since been reported to be sensitive to the toxic effects of TNF (Shalaby *et al.*, 1989a).

The toxicity of TNF appeared to be dose related. At 1 μg/mouse, there were occasional foci of necrosis of the mucosa in the small intestine. This necrosis was observed primarily at the tips of the villi (Remick *et al.*, 1987; Kunkel *et al.*, 1989). At the higher dose of 10 μg, there were more severe changes. TNF-treated animals had blunting of the villi, with frank necrosis of the mucosa at the tips of the villi. These changes have been described as though a lawn mower had moved down the lumen of the small bowel, destroying mucosa and shearing off the tips of the villi. These changes are highly reproducible. In several "blind" experiments, the pathologist (DGR) was always able to determine those animals treated with rHuTNF. Also, at the 10-μg dose, there was some evidence of scattered epithelial damage to the large intestine, although the changes were not nearly as dramatic as those in the small intestine.

C. Ultrastructural Changes and Vascular Leak

The small intestine was examined by electron microscopy, to confirm the light microscopy changes and to provide further insight into the mechanism of damage. Figure 3 shows an electron micrograph of the small intestine from an animal sacrificed 2 hr after injection of 10 μg or rHuTNF. The surface epithelium demonstrated necrosis of the cells, with some showing almost complete loss of the cytoplasm. The lamina propria was expanded by inflammatory cells. Figure 4 shows extravasated neutrophils. Other areas (not shown) had leakage of red cells, and extrusion of granules from the Paneth cells. Animals receiving normal saline alone never displayed any alterations.

We turned our attention to the vasculature of the small intestine, to determine if the observed toxicity could possibly be explained by disruption of the blood vessels. Severe endothelial cell damage could be discerned in the vessels at the base of the lamina propria, illustrated in Fig. 5. There was extensive blebbing of the endothelial cell luminal surface and vacuolization of the cytoplasm. Gap formation between the endothelial cells was present, with exposed basement membrane. The disruption and destruction of the

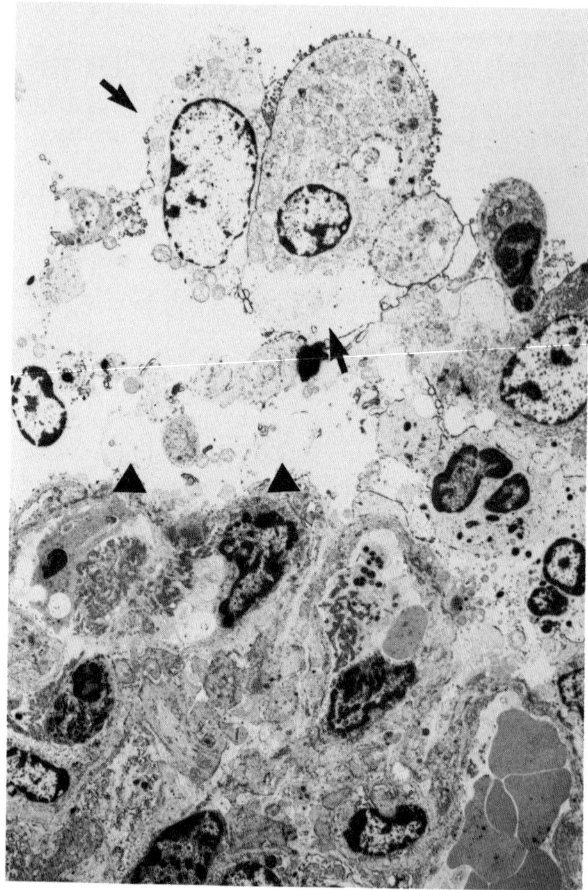

Fig. 3. Low-power electron micrograph of TNF-induced small bowel epithelial damage. TNF (10 μg) was injected intravenously into CBA/J mice and the small intestine was examined 2 hr later. At low power, there is destruction of the epithelial cells with vacuolization and loss of cytoplasm (arrows). The submucosa also exhibits edema (triangles) ($\times$2000).

endothelial cells provides an explanation for the leakage of the inflammatory cells and red blood cells into the lamina propria.

The leakage of fluid into the small intestine was quantitated by assessing the extravasation of ^{125}I-labeled albumin from the vasculature into the organs. For these experiments, ^{125}I-labeled albumin was injected along with the rHuTNF and the animals were sacrificed 2 hr later. Blood was collected and the heart perfused with normal saline, and each organ was removed and counted in a γ counter. The counts per minute (cpm) from all of the organs, and the blood, were totaled and the results expressed as a percentage of the

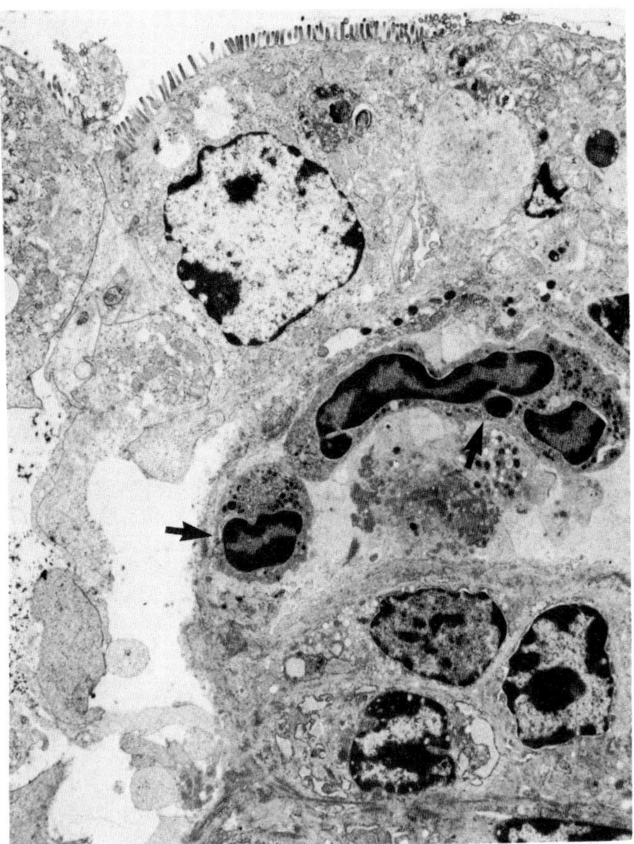

Fig. 4. High-power electron micrograph of TNF-induced small bowel epithelial damage. TNF (10 μg) was injected intravenously into CBA/J mice and the small intestine was examined 2 hr later. This area shows extravasation of two neutrophils (arrows) outside of the blood vessels, where they lie just beneath the epithelial cell layer ($\times$3700).

total recovered cpm. Using this sensitive approach, increasing leakage of fluid with increasing amounts of TNF was documented into the small intestine at the 1- and 10-μg doses. At the 10-μg dose there was also evidence of leakage into the large intestine. None of the other organs showed evidence of developing a vascular leak (Remick *et al.,* 1987).

D. Comparison to Previous Experiments

Other investigators have evaluated the toxicity of rHuTNF injection into experimental animals. Tracey *et al.* (1986) were the first to report that

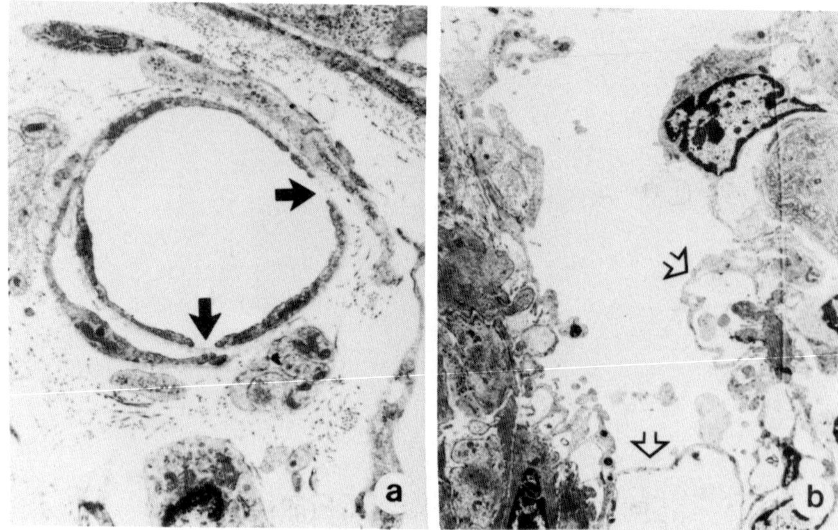

Fig. 5. Ultrastructural examination of TNF-induced vascular damage. rHuTNF (10 μg) was injected intravenously and the vasculature of the small bowel was examined 2 hr later. (a) The endothelium shows severe damage with gap formation and exposed basement membrane (arrows; ×11,500). (b) Other areas disclose endothelial cell damage with marked blebbing of the luminal surface (arrows; ×3050).

rHuTNF would cause widespread organ injury. However, the doses used in his study were much greater than we employed. The difference in the dosage accounts for the less severe injury observed in our study. This group has also shown that rHuTNF will induce shock and organ injury in beagle dogs, with pulmonary, renal, and adrenal damage (Tracey *et al.,* 1987b).

Shalaby also looked at the organ injury with TNF, and documented that the uterus was particularly sensitive to necrosis (Shalaby *et al.,* 1989a). Talmadge *et al.* (1987) also found that rHuTNF would synergize with interferon-γ to induce foci of coagulative necrosis in the lungs, liver, gastrointestinal tract, testes, uterus, and bone marrow. The synergistic toxic effects of TNF with other cytokines has also been described for interleukin-1 (Waage and Espevik, 1988).

IV. ADDITIONAL TOXICITY OF TNF

A. High-Dose TNF

Given the documented, widespread toxicity of higher doses of TNF, we investigated the spectrum of organ injury observed after intravenous injection of 10 or 100 μg of rHuTNF. These experiments were very limited, and involved only three animals because it was difficult to obtain sufficient

Table I. Lung Injury Induced by TNF

	Cells per high-power field (mean ± SEM)	
TNF (μg)	Red blood cells	Neutrophils
Control	5.2 ± 0.4	3.8 ± 0.3
10	2.7 ± 0.3	19 ± 0.6
100	46 ± 6	23 ± 1

recombinant material for more extensive studies. Also, the experiments were performed to confirm other investigators' work, and not to provide additional insight into the toxicology of TNF. Organs were examined ultra-structurally 2 hr after intravenous injection, in order to maximize the possibility of detecting tissue damage. As in the previous study, the 10-μg dose caused damage to the small intestine. The changes were similar to those described above, and included endothelial cell damage. At the 100-μg dose, there was also damage to the kidneys with vacuolization of the tubular epithelium.

The lungs showed more severe damage, with increased interstitial edema, endothelial cell damage, and leakage of platelets, inflammatory cells, red blood cells, and fibrin into the alveolar spaces. Table I shows the results of a morphometric analysis of this damage. In a blind study, 100 high-powered fields (hpf; ×40 objective) were examined from each of the experimental animals. The data show a significant increase in the number of red blood cells/hpf, and a significant increase in the number of neutrophils/hpf.

B. Dose-Dependent Toxicity of TNF

These data suggest that rHuTNF has a dose-dependent toxic effect *in vivo*. At the lowest doses, peripheral blood alterations occur, with relative lymphopenia and neutrophilia developing at a dose of 0.01 μg. Absolute neutrophilia occurs at 0.1 μg, and absolute lymphopenia at 1 μg. Damage to the small bowel may be seen with 1 μg, but is well developed at 10 μg. At a dose of 100 μg, there is slight renal tubular damage and extensive pulmonary injury.

V. COMPARISON OF ENDOGENOUS AND EXOGENOUS TNF

A. Endogenous Production of TNF

As stated previously, our working hypothesis is that endotoxin or LPS induces TNF and the TNF in turn causes the altered pathophysiology. To prove this hypothesis, several experiments must be performed. The first group of experiments would need to demonstrate that after administration of LPS, TNF is produced. Given the large numbers of publications on this matter, there can be no doubt that injection of LPS results in significant TNF production. This has been shown at the level of both biologically active material (Shalaby *et al.,* 1989b), as well as by material that can be detected by ELISA (Nguyen *et al.,* 1990). Additionally, mRNA coding for mouse TNF may be detected after injection of LPS (DeForge *et al.,* 1990; Remick *et al.,* 1987, 1990). Another group of experiments is to inject the recombinant, purified TNF and document that changes occur similar to those observed after injection of LPS, which has been extensively reviewed in the preceding section.

B. Peripheral Blood Changes

Peripheral blood alterations have been described after injection of LPS (Kunkel *et al.,* 1989; Remick *et al.,* 1990). We closely examined the changes in the percentages of lymphocytes and neutrophils after injection of either 1 μg of rHuTNF or 10 μg of LPS in CBA/J mice. For these experiments, the mice were previously primed by the intraperitoneal injection of complete Freund's adjuvant, because prior immunization with bacillus Calmette–Guérin (BCG) has been classically used to heighten the TNF response to the LPS challenge (Carswell *et al.,* 1975). It should be noted that the rHuTNF was injected intravenously, whereas the LPS was injected intraperitoneally. Figure 6 demonstrates the close similarity of the changes in the peripheral blood constituents, both the magnitude of the changes as well as the kinetics of the change. Both TNF and LPS induced a relative neutrophilia and lymphopenia, with maximum changes occurring by 2–4 hr. The LPS peripheral blood changes appeared to be more long-lasting, because there was no evidence of return to normal values even 28 hr after LPS challenge. The injection of the LPS resulted in the induction of about 1000 U of TNF, i.e., 45 ng of endogenous TNF.

C. Small Bowel Damage

Intestinal damage has been documented after injection of LPS (Lillehei and Maclean, 1958) and the studies described above showed severe injury preferentially targeted to the intestine. After injection of the LPS, virtually all mice become lethargic and develop piloerection. Watery diarrhea invariably occurs, and a blind evaluation allows an observer to determine quickly which mice were treated with LPS. Figure 7 shows the histology of the small intestine 2 hr after injection of 10 μg of rHuTNF, or 4 hr after injection of 10 μg of LPS. The histologic alterations are similar and consist of damage to

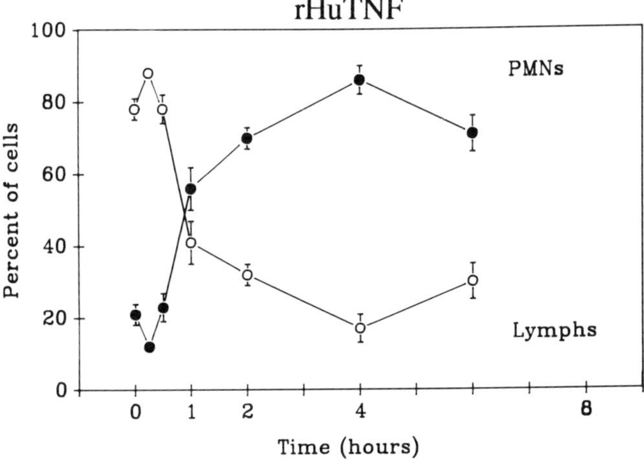

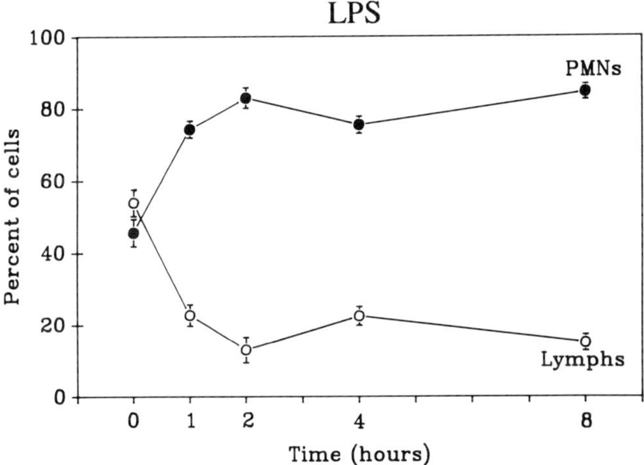

Fig. 6. Peripheral blood alterations after either LPS or rHuTNF challenge. rHuTNF was injected intravenously at 1 μg/mouse; 10 μg of LPS was injected into Freund's adjuvant-primed mice. Both agents induced a rapid lymphopenia and neutrophilia, with clearly demonstrable changes present by 1 hr.

the epithelium on the tips of the villi. The mucosa in this region is disrupted and the cells are necrotic. The microscopic sections were taken from similar locations in the bowel, and also demonstrate some slight shortening of the length of the villi. Functional changes have also been described in the intestine after injection of TNF (van Lanschott *et al.,* 1990). Additional investigations have closely looked at the relationship between the induction

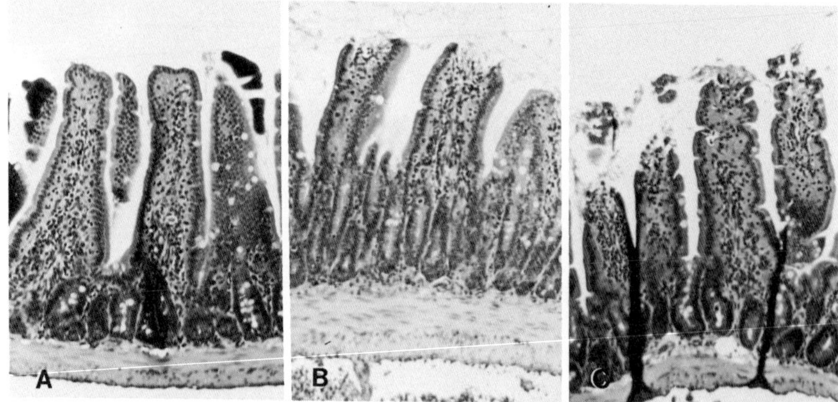

Fig. 7. Histology of TNF- and LPS-induced small bowel damage. CBA/J mice were injected with vehicle alone (a), with 10 μg of LPS into Freund's-primed mice (b), or with 10 μg of rHuTNF (c). The control mice have tall, intact villi with no disruption of the surface epithelium (a). After 4 hr postinjection of LPS, there is slight shortening of the villi, with necrosis of the mucosal epithelial cells at the tips of the villi (b). Similar changes are observed 2 hr postinjection of 10 μg of rHuTNF (c). All micrographs are at the same magnification.

of platelet-activating factor, tumor necrosis factor, and intestinal injury (Sun and Hsueh, 1988; Hsueh and Sun, 1989)

D. Vascular Permeability Changes

Because rHuTNF caused an actual increase in vascular permeability in the small intestine, we investigated whether the histologic damage observed after LPS would also result in leakage of plasma proteins into the small bowel. LPS induced extravasation of [125]labeled albumin into the small bowel, similar to that observed with rHuTNF. Figure 8 shows that either rHuTNF or LPS causes a similar change. These data confirm the histologic impression of damage to the small intestine.

E. Pulmonary Changes

TNF has been implicated in pulmonary damage, because patients with adult respiratory distress syndrome have TNF present in their bronchoalveolar lavage fluid (Millar *et al.,* 1989), and injection of TNF induces pulmonary injury (Stephens *et al.,* 1988). After injection of LPS there is rapid sequestration of neutrophils in the pulmonary vasculature (Remick *et al.,* 1990), although no clear-cut injury could be documented. Thus both TNF and LPS will induce neutrophils to lodge in the lung, although the high dose of TNF also apparently caused them to induce damage.

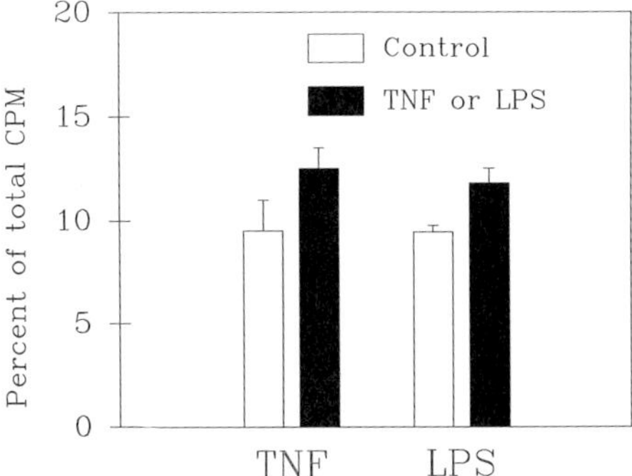

Fig. 8. Vascular permeability changes after injection of rHuTNF or LPS. Leakage of ^{125}I-labeled albumin is observed when mice are treated with either purified recombinant TNF, or endogenous TNF is produced by the LPS challenge. For TNF, the permeability was determined 2 hr postintravenous injection; the endogenous TNF was determined 8 hr postintraperitoneal LPS challenge. Each data point is the mean ± SEM for three to five mice.

VI. INHIBITION OF TOXICITY WITH ANTI-TNF ANTIBODY

A. Antibody Specificity

Demonstrating that TNF is elevated after LPS injection and that both compounds induce similar pathology does not prove a cause-and-effect relationship. The most rigorous evidence for this would be to inhibit the activity of TNF *in vivo* with a specific antibody. We prepared such an antibody by immunizing rabbits with purified, recombinant murine TNF (Remick *et al.,* 1990). This antibody will completely neutralize 10 U of mouse TNF at a dilution of 1 : 25,000 in a standard LM cytolytic assay, and will detect as little as 100 pg of murine TNF in a Western blot analysis at a dilution of 1 : 1,000,000. Figure 9 shows that the antibody has specificity for TNF, with no cross-reactivity with IL-1-α or -β. The antibody also does not cross-react with LPS, because treatment with the antibody did not inhibit the ability of LPS to induce IL-1 production.

B. *In Vivo* Inhibition of TNF Biological Activity

CBA/J mice were treated with complete Freund's adjuvant, and 2 weeks later were injected with 10 μg of LPS along with a 1 : 100 dilution of the antibody. Figure 10 shows that this antibody is able to completely inhibit the TNF activity in the ascites fluid harvested 1 hr after LPS stimulation. The control animals received a 1 : 100 dilution of normal rabbit serum and showed production of TNF. We have obtained similar data using nonprimed mice with the antibody, wherein it is able to prevent completely the appearance of TNF in the plasma after a lethal LPS challenge.

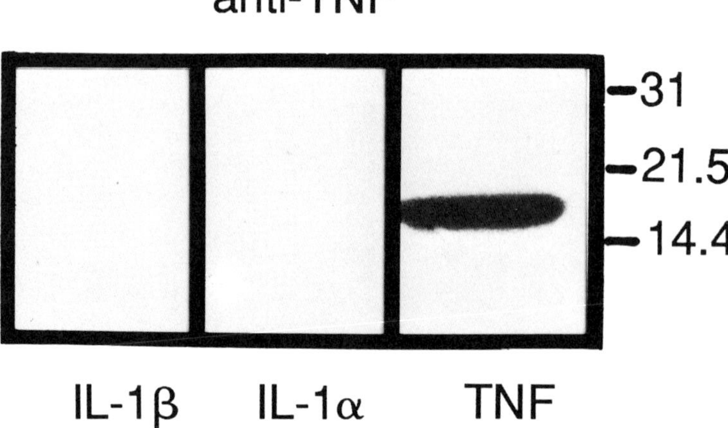

Fig. 9. Western blot analysis of specificity of anti-TNF antibody. The indicated purified, recombinant cytokines (100 ng) were subjected to polyacrylamide gel electrophoresis and then Western blot analysis using the anti-TNF antibody. The antibody recognized only the TNF, with no apparent cross-reactivity to interleukin-1-α or -β.

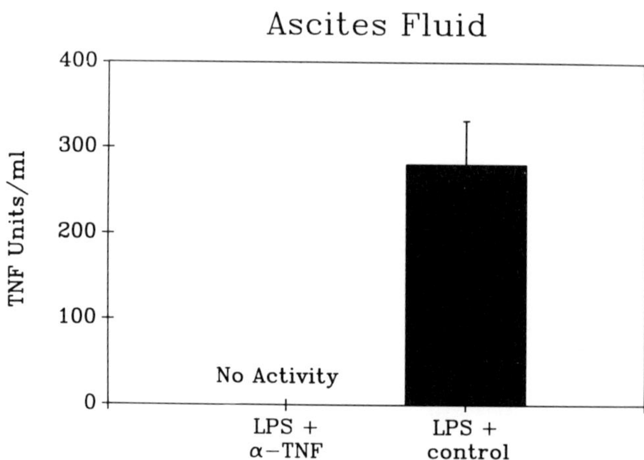

Fig. 10. Ability of anti-TNF antibody to inhibit TNF biological activity *in vivo*. CBA/J mice were primed with complete Freund's adjuvant and injected 2 weeks later with 10 μg of LPS mixed with either control rabbit serum or anti-TNF antiserum. At the peak of TNF biological activity (1 hr later), ascites fluid was harvested and analyzed for TNF biological activity. Mice treated with anti-TNF antiserum had no detectable TNF. The values are the mean $\pm$ SEM for five mice.

C. Reduction in Altered Pathophysiology

We have described several changes observed after injection of LPS or TNF into mice. Several of these changes are directly comparable, i.e., the peripheral blood changes, the damage to the small intestine, and neutrophil sequestration in the lung. Using a specific anti-TNF antibody, we have carefully examined the role of TNF in pathophysiologic alterations occurring at the 1-hr time point. Administration of the antibody could completely prevent the peripheral blood changes (Remick *et al.,* 1990). It must be mentioned that only the 1-hr time point post-LPS injection was examined, and it is possible that other cytokines participate at later time points. The antibody preparation was also able to inhibit, but not completely prevent, neutrophil accumulation in the lung. Again, only the 1-hr time point was examined.

VII. SUMMARY

Work from several laboratories has documented that TNF is toxic *in vivo.* The data are sufficiently compelling that there is little doubt that this small peptide mediator can induce altered pathophysiology and tissue damage if injected in large quantities. Whereas injection of high-dose, exogenous rHu-TNF results in toxicity, and the production of very high levels in lethal septic shock is detrimental, the exact role of this molecule in inflammation is yet to be defined completely. At low, physiologic levels, TNF may be a necessary component required to orchestrate an effective immune response to a successful resolution. Several works have shown that inhibition of TNF with specific antibodies in models of bacterial infection can decrease survival (Havell, 1987; Echtenacher *et al.,* 1990). Clearly, further work must be done to resolve the issue of the exact role of TNF in organ injury during septic shock.

Acknowledgments

This work was supported in part by National Institutes of Health Grants HL32127, HL31963, HL35276, HL39339, and GM44198, and by a Grant-in-Aid from the American Heart Association of Michigan.

References

Beutler, B., Milsark, I. W., and Cerami, A. C. (1985a). *Science* **229,** 869–871.
Beutler, B. A., Milsark, I. W., and Cerami, A. (1985b). *J. Immunol.* **135,** 3972–3977.
Carswell, E. A., Old, L. J., Kassel, R. L., Green, S., Fiore, N., and Williamson, B. (1975). *Proc. Natl. Acad. Sci. U.S.A.* **72,** 3666–3670.
Chong, K. T., and Huston, M. (1987). *J. Infect. Dis.* **156,** 713–719.

Debets, J. M., Kampmeijer, R., van der Linden, M. P., Buurman, A., and van der Linden, C. J. (1989). *Crit. Care Med.* **17**, 489–494.

DeForge, L. E., Nguyen, D. T., Kunkel, S. L., and Remick, D. G. (1990). *J. Lab. Clin. Med.* **116**, 429–438.

Echtenacher, B., Falk, W., Mannel, D. N., and Krammer, P. H. (1990). *J. Immunol.* **145**, 3762–3766.

Havell, E. A. (1987). *J. Immunol.* **139**, 4225–4231.

Hinshaw, L. B., Tekamp-Olson, P., Chang, A. C., Lee, P. A., Taylor, B., Jr., Murray, C. K., Peer, G. T., Emerson, T. E., Jr., Passey, B., and Kuo, G. C. (1990). *Circ. Shock* **30**, 279–292.

Hsueh, W., and Sun, X. M. (1989). *Adv. Prostaglandin Thromboxane Leukotriene Res.* **19**, 363–366.

Kunkel., S. L., Remick, D. G., Strieter, R. M., and Larrick, J. W. (1989). *Crit. Rev. Immunol.* **9**, 93–117.

Lahdevirta, J., Maury, C. P., Teppo, A. M., and Repo, H. (1988). *Am. J. Med.* **85**, 289–291.

Levine, B., Kalman, J., Mayer, L., Fillit, H. M., and Packer, M. (1990). *N. Engl. J. Med.* **323**, 236–241.

Lillehei, R. C., and Maclean, L. D. (1958). *Ann. Surg.* **148**, 513–521.

Marks, J. D., Marks, C. B., Luce, J. M., Montgomery, A. B., Turner, J., Metz, C. A., and Murray, J. F. (1990). *Am. Rev. Respir. Dis.* **141**, 94–97.

Mathison, J. C., Wolfson, E., and Ulevitch, R. J. (1988). *J. Clin. Invest.* **81**, 1925–1937.

Maury, C. P., and Teppo, A. M. (1987). *J. Exp. Med.* **166**, 1132–1137.

Michie, H. R., Manogue, K. R., Spriggs, D. R., Revhaug, A., O'Dwyer, S., Dinarello, C. A., Cerami, A., Wolff, S. M., and Wilmore, D. W. (1988). *N. Engl. J. Med.* **318**, 1481–1486.

Millar, A. B., Foley, N. M., Singer, M., Johnson, N. M., Meager, A., and Rook, G. A. (1989). *Lancet* **ii**, 712–714.

Neter, E., Gorzynski, E. A., Westphal, O., and Luderitz, O. (1958). *J. Immunol.* **80**, 66–72.

Nguyen, D. T., Eskandari, M. K., DeForge, L. E., Raiford, C. L., Strieter, R. M., Kunkel, S. L., and Remick, D. G. (1990). *J. Immunol.* **144**, 3822–3828.

Playfair, J. H., de Souza, J. B., and Taverne, J. (1982). *Clin. Exp. Immunol.* **47**, 753–755.

Remick, D. G. (1991). *Lab. Invest.* **65**, 259–261.

Remick, D. G., Larrick, J., and Kunkel, S. L. (1986). *Biochem. Biophys. Res. Commun.* **141**, 818–824.

Remick, D. G., Kunkel, R. G., Larrick, J. W., and Kunkel, S. L. (1987). *Lab. Invest.* **56**, 583–590.

Remick, D. G., Strieter, R.M., Lynch, J. P., Nguyen, D., Eskandari, M., and Kunkel, S. L. (1989). *Lab. Invest.* **60**, 766–771.

Remick, D. G., Strieter, R. M., Eskandari, M. K., Nguyen, D. T., Genord, M. A., Raiford, C. L., and Kunkel, S. L. (1990). *Am. J. Pathol.* **136**, 49–60.

Saxne, T., Palladino, M. A., Jr., Heinegard, D., Talal, N., and Wollheim, F. A. (1988). *Arthritis Rheum.* **31**, 1041–1045.

Scuderi, P., Sterling, K. E., Lam, K. S., Finley, P. R., Ryan, K. J., Ray, C. G., Petersen, E., Slymen, D. J., and Salmon, S. E. (1986). *Lancet* **ii**, 1364–1365.

Shalaby, M. R., Laegreid, W. W., Ammann, A. J., and Liggitt, H. D. (1989a). *Lab. Invest.* **61**, 564–570.

Shalaby, M. R., Waage, A., Aarden, L., and Expevik, T. (1989b). *Clin. Immunol. Immunopathol.* **53**, 488–498.

Spriggs, D. R., Sherman, M. L., Michie, H., Arthur, K. A., Immura, K., Wilmore, D., Frei, D. E., III, and Kafe, D. W. (1988). *J. Natl. Cancer Inst.* **80**, 1039–1044.

Stephens, K. E., Ishizaka, A., Larrick, J. W., and Raffin, T. A. (1988). *Am. Rev. Respir. Dis.* **137**, 1364–1370.

Sun, X. M., and Hsueh, W. (1988). *J. Clin. Invest.* **81**, 1328–1331.

Talmadge, J. E., Bowersox, O., Tribble, H., Lee, S. H., Shepard, M., and Liggitt, D. (1987). *Am. J. Pathol.* **128**, 410–425.

Tracey, K. J., Beutler, B., Lowry, S. F., Merryweather, J., Wolpe, Milsark, I. W., Hariri, R. J., Fahey, T. J., III, Zentella, A., Albert, J. D., Shires, G. T., and Cerami, A. (1986). *Science* **234**, 470–474.

Tracey, K. J., Fong, Y., Hesse, D. G., Manogue, K. R., Lee, A. T., Kuo, G. C., Lowry, S. F., and Cerami, A. (1987a). *Nature (London)* **330**, 662–664.

Tracey, K. J., Lowry, S. F., Fahey, T. J., III, Albert, J. D., Fong, Y., Hesse, D., Beutler, B., Manogue, K. R., Calvano, S., Wei, H., *et al.* (1987b). *Surg. Gynecol. Obstet.* **164**, 415–422.

Ulich, T. R., del Castillo, J., Keys, M., Granger, G. A., and Ni, R. X. (1987). *J. Immunol.* **139**, 3406–3415.

Ulich, T. R., del Castillo, J., Ni, R. X., Bikhazi, N., and Calvin, L. (1989). *J. Leukocyte Biol.* **45**, 155–167.

van Lanschot, J. J., Mealy, K., and Wilmore, D. W. (1990). *Ann. Surg.* **212**, 663–670.

Waage, A. (1987). *Clin. Immunol. Immunopathol.* **45**, 348–355.

Waage, A., and Espevik, T. (1988). *J. Exp. Med.* **167**, 1987–1992.

Waage, A., Halstensen, A., and Espevik, T. (1987). *Lancet* **1**, 355–357.

Watson, J., Kelly, K., Largen, M., and Taylor, B. A. (1978). *J. Immunol.* **120**, 422–424.

In Vitro and *in Vivo* Activity and Pathophysiology of Human Interleukin-8 and Related Peptides

Roland Zwahlen
Institut für Tierpathologie
Universität Bern
CH-3001 Bern 9, Switzerland

Alfred Walz
Theodor Kocher Institut
Universität Bern
CH-3001 Bern 9, Switzerland

Antal Rot
Sandoz Forschungsinstitut
A-1235 Vienna, Austria

I. INTRODUCTION

Acute inflammation is characterized by leukocyte emigration and plasma exudation from blood vessels into diseased tissues. Systematic studies of phagocyte recruitment and activation have become possible with the identification of a number of endogenous and exogenous chemoattractants, such as bacterial-derived *N*-formylmethionyl peptides (fMLPs) (Schiffmann *et al.,* 1975; Rot *et al.,* 1987), fragments from activated complement (C5a) (Fernandez *et al.,* 1978), and the two bioactive lipids, platelet-activating factor (PAF) and leukotriene B_4 (LTB$_4$) (Shaw *et al.,* 1981; Ford Hutchinson *et al.,* 1980). Recently, three low-molecular-weight peptide factors with neutrophil-stimulating properties were identified. These are (1) neutrophil-activating peptide-1/interleukin-8 (NAP-1/IL-8), a peptide originally isolated from the conditioned media of stimulated human mononuclear cells (Walz *et al.,* 1987; Schroeder *et al.,* 1987; Yoshimura *et al.,* 1987), (2) the platelet-derived neutrophil-activating peptide-2 (NAP-2) (Walz and Baggiolini, 1989), and (3) GRO-α, a peptide originally reported to stimulate melanoma cell growth (Anisowicz *et al.,* 1987; Richmond and Thomas, 1988; Moser *et al.,* 1990). IL-8, NAP-2, and GRO-α belong to a subfamily of small peptides (8–10 kDa) containing four conserved cysteine residues, the first two spaced by one amino acid (CXC). Other prominent members of this family, lacking neutrophil-activating properties, are platelet factor-4 and connective tissue-activating peptide III (precursor for NAP-2) (Walz, 1991; Oppenheim *et al.,* 1991). A related subfamily contains peptides that are chemotactic for monocytes and lymphocytes, such as monocyte chemotactic peptide-1 (MCP-1), regulated on activation, normal T expressed and secreted (RANTES), macrophage inflammatory protein-1α and -1β (MIP-1α, MIP-1β), and others (Schall, 1991), all of which have the first cysteine residues adjacent (CC).

Here we review the induction, formation, and *in vitro* biological effects of neutrophil-activating peptides. In addition we summarize the effects of IL-8 following systemic and peripheral application in laboratory animals, and of GRO-α and NAP-2 following injection into the rat skin.

II. INDUCTION AND FORMATION

IL-8 was originally isolated from culture supernatants of stimulated human blood mononuclear cells. Subsequently it has been demonstrated that IL-8 is induced and secreted from many different cells, such as monocytes, alveolar macrophages, lymphocytes, fibroblasts, endothelial cells, epithelial cells, keratinocytes, synovial cells, and others (Baggiolini *et al.,* in press). Whereas the proinflammatory cytokines tumor necrosis factor (TNF), IL-1α, and IL-1β are inducers for IL-8 in most of the cell types, other stimuli have a more limited range of activity: lipopolysaccharide (LPS), for example, induces IL-8 production only in phagocytes and endothelial cells.

GRO-α was originally described as a product of transformed cells and was termed melanoma growth-stimulatory activity (MGSA). It was later found to be expressed and released by several types of normal cells, such as monocytes, neutrophils, and fibroblasts, as well as endothelial, epithelial, and synovial cells. GRO is expressed under conditions that yield high levels of IL-8, e.g., exposure to IL-1, TNF, or LPS. Three closely related genes encoding for GRO-α, GRO-β (MIP-2α), and Gro-γ (MIP-2β) have been identified (Haskill *et al.,* 1990; Tekamp-Olson *et al.,* 1990). The expression of the different genes and the biological functions of the corresponding peptides will have to be clarified.

The cell source and formation of NAP-2 differs from that of IL-8 and GRO. NAP-2 is formed by specific proteolytic cleavage from precursors contained in the α granules of platelets. On platelet activation, the precursors platelet basic protein and connective tissue-activating peptide III (CTAP-III) are released from the platelets and are processed by monocyte or neutrophil proteases to yield NAP-2. Cathepsin G, a protease contained in monocytes and neutrophils, was shown to selectively cleave CTAP-III into NAP-2 (Walz and Baggiolini, 1990; Car *et al.,* 1991).

III. BIOLOGICAL ACTIVITIES *in Vitro*

A. Activities on Neutrophils

IL-8, NAP-2, and GRO-α are potent activators of human neutrophils *in vitro.* They induce shape change, chemotaxis, a rise in intracellular free calcium, respiratory burst, exocytosis of azurophil and specific granules, and secretory vesicles (Table I) (Baggiolini *et al.,* in press). In addition, it was demonstrated that IL-8 up-regulates complement receptors 1 and 3 (CR1 and CR3, or CD11b and CD18) on the surface of human neutrophils and also increases the binding capacity of CR3 for fibrinogen-coated surfaces and endothelial cell monolayers (Detmers *et al.,* 1990; Paccaud *et al.,* 1990; Carveth *et al.,* 1989). The relative potency of the three agonists varies considerably among

Table I. Neutrophil Responses to IL-8, NAP-2, and GRO-α

	IL-8	NAP-2	GRO-α
Ca^{2+} rise	+++	+++	+++
Chemotaxis[a]	+++	+++	+++
Chemotaxis[b]	+++	+	n.d.
Exocytosis	+++	++	++
Respiratory burst	++	+	+
Polymorphonuclear cell infiltration (rabbit)	+++	+++	+++
Polymorphonuclear cell infiltration (rat)	+++	+	+++

[a] Nitrocellulose membranes, method as described by Schroeder *et al.* (1987).
[b] Polycarbonate membranes, method as described by Leonard *et al.* (1991b). GRO-α not determined (n.d.).

the different neutrophil responses. IL-8 was equipotent to NAP-2 and GRO-α as a stimulus of cytosolic free calcium changes and chemotaxis using nitrocellulose membranes (Walz *et al.*, 1989). However, IL-8 was considerably more potent as a stimulus of exocytosis and respiratory burst (Walz *et al.*, 1989, 1991a), and of chemotaxis using polycarbonate membranes (Leonard *et al.*, 1991b). Human IL-8 induces *in vitro* chemotaxis in neutrophils of rabbit, rat, mouse, guinea pig, goat, dog, pig, monkey, and chicken; however, its potency for the neutrophils of these species varies broadly (Rot, 1991).

B. Activities on Other Leukocytes

IL-8 was reported to be chemotactic for basophils (Leonard *et al.*, 1990) and to induce histamine release only after pretreatment with IL-3 (Dahinden *et al.*, 1989). The chemotactic response of basophils to IL-8 is enhanced by IL-3 pretreatment (A. Rot, unpublished observations). IL-8 does not induce chemotaxis in monocytes and eosinophils (Leonard *et al.*, 1990), but eosinophils become responsive on IL-3 pretreatment (Waringa *et al.*, 1991). Human monocytes respond to IL-8 and GRO-α, but not to NAP-2, with a concentration-dependent intracellular calcium rise and, when primed with concanavalin A (ConA), with a respiratory burst signal (Walz *et al.*, 1991a). IL-8 has been reported to attract human lymphocytes *in vitro* (Bacon *et al.*, 1989), in particular, T cells (Leonard *et al.*, 1990; Larsen *et al.*, 1989).

IV. BIOLOGICAL ACTIVITIES *in Vivo*

A. Methods

1. Inflammatory Agents

Recombinant human IL-8 (Lindley *et al.*, 1988) was kept at 400 μg/ml in 50 mM 2-(N-morpholino)ethanesulfonic acid, 0.43 M NaCl, pH 6.5, and diluted shortly before use with pyrogen-free saline (PFS) to 10^{-9}, 10^{-10}, and 10^{-11} mol per 50 μl. Platelet-activating factor (PAF, 1-O-hexadecyl-*sn*-glycero-3-phosphorylcholine; Bachem AG) was diluted to 10^{-9} mol per 50 μl in PFS containing 0.1% bovine serum albumin (BSA). Endotoxin (*Escherichia coli,* serotype O55:B5, assumed MW 12,000; Sigma) was dissolved in PFS to a dilution of 10^{-13} mol per 50 μl. Highly purified NAP-2 (Walz and Baggiolini, 1989) was diluted with PFS to yield 10^{-9}, 10^{-10}, and 10^{-11} mol per 50 μl. Synthetic GRO-α was obtained from Dr. I. Clark-Lewis (University of Vancouver, Canada) and was similarly diluted.

For intradermal injection, male Wistar rats weighing 180–200 g were used. The hairs on the back were clipped short the day before the experiment; 50 μl of the chemoattractants and of pyrogen-free saline were injected intradermally using 26-gauge hypodermic needles and tuberculin syringes.

Injection was performed under light ether anesthesia. After respective time intervals, the animals were killed with an overdose of ether.

For systemic application, recombinant human IL-8 was injected intravenously into Chinchilla rabbits. Three injection protocols were used: (1) Four rabbits received a single intravenous (i.v.) bolus injection of 100 μg of IL-8. Pyrogen-free phosphate-buffered saline [PBS; LPS $<$ 1 pg/ml, when tested in the limulus aemobocide lysate (LAL) assay] served as a control. Two rabbits were sacrificed 3 hr after injection. Blood samples were taken periodically from the remaining animals to perform absolute and differential leukocyte counts. (2) Two rabbits received three i.v. injections of 100 μg IL-8 at 1-hr intervals. Control animals received three injections with PBS. Animals were sacrificed 3 hr after the last injection. (3) Four rabbits received one daily i.v. injection of IL-8 (40 μg/kg) during five consecutive days. PBS served as a control. Two animals were sacrificed 3 hr after, and two animals 2 weeks after, the last injection. Routine histological examination of 4% buffered formaldehyde-fixed parenchymal organs was performed.

2. Histology for Intradermal Injections

After excision the skin was fixed in 4% buffered formaldehyde. Full-thickness skin samples were cut out of each site, embedded in paraffin, processed routinely, and stained with hematoxylin and eosin. Neutrophil infiltrates within the skin were evaluated semiquantitatively (Munro *et al.,* 1989). Coded samples were scored blindly for the intensity of extravascular cellular accumulation using set scales for neutrophils. Granulocyte accumulation was assessed separately in the upper dermis, reaching from epithelium to the deepest adnexal structures, and in the lower dermis reaching from the deepest adnexal structures to the panniculus carnosus. Scores (see Fig. 1)

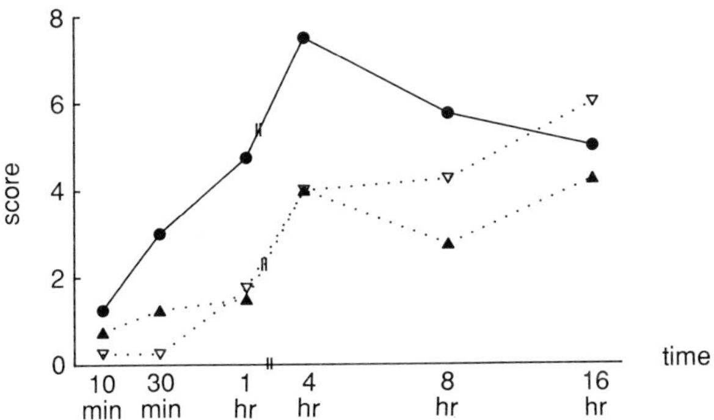

Fig. 1. Inflammatory score after a single intradermal injection of different agonists in rats. Comparison between values of sites treated with 10^{-9} mol IL-8 ($\bullet$, n = 4), 10^{-9} mol platelet-activating factor ($\blacktriangle$, n = 4), and 10^{-13} mol endotoxin ($\triangle$, n = 4).

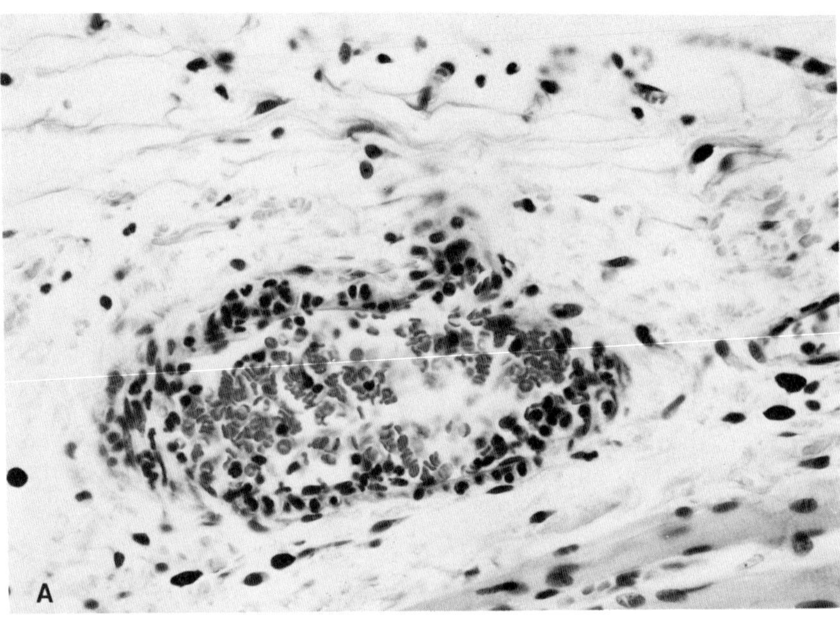

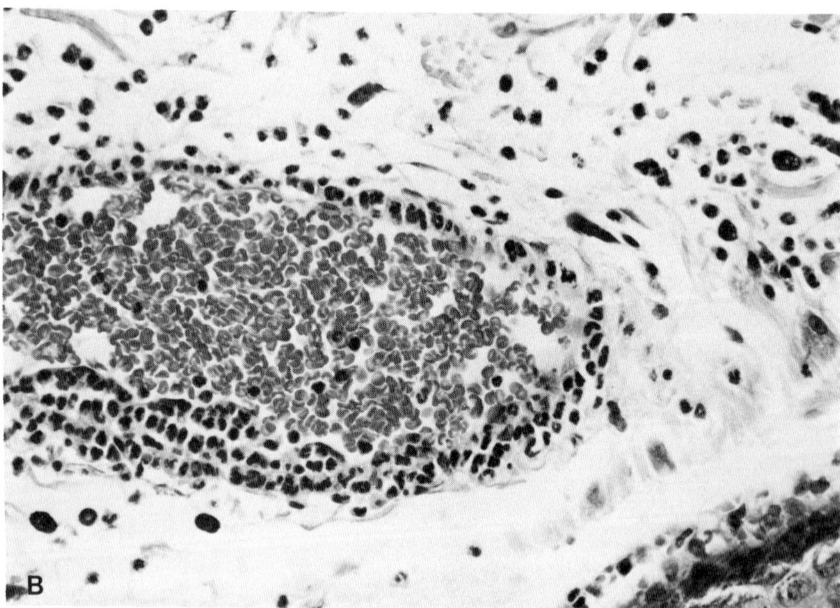

Fig. 2. Rat lower dermis after injection of 10^{-9} mol of IL-8; cross-section of a venule. (a) At 30 min after injection; accumulation of neutrophils within the vessel wall; few neutrophils present in the perivascular area. (b) At 60 min after injection; an excessive number of neutrophils is accumulated in the subendothelial area and within the vessel wall; a moderate number of neutrophils is in the perivascular area. (c) At 4 hr after

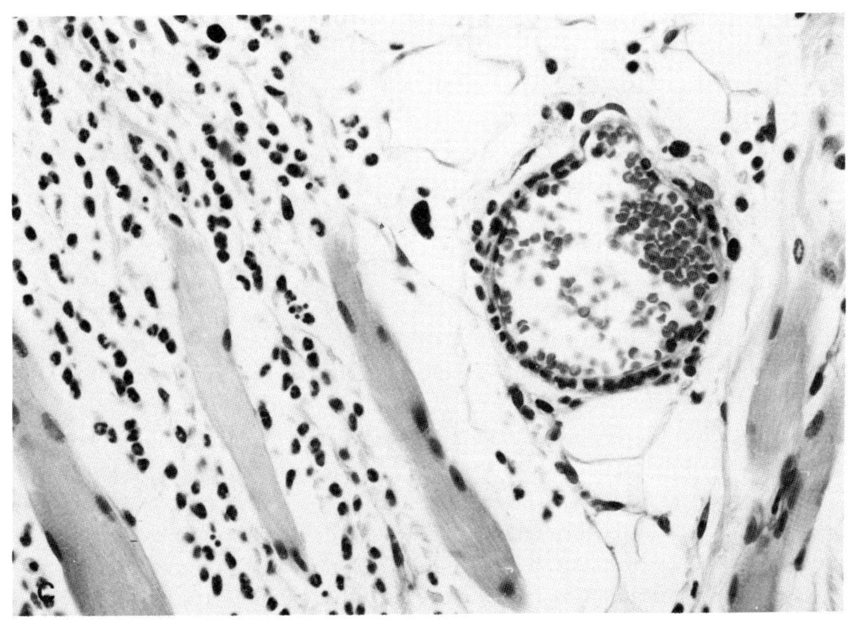

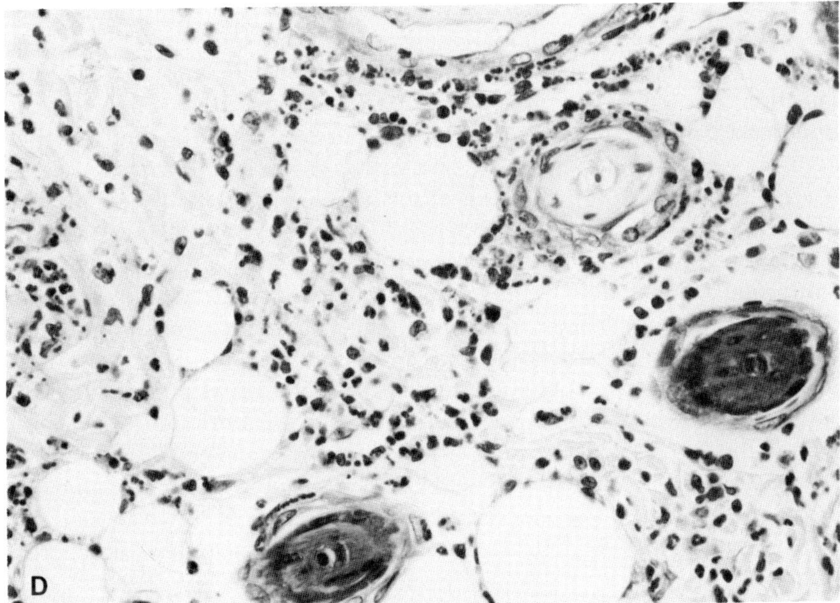

injection; a large number of neutrophils is present between muscle fibers of the panniculus carnosus and a moderate number of neutrophils is still present in the venular wall. (d) At 16 hr after injection; a large number of diffusely scattered neutrophils is still present in the interstitium; they demonstrate distinct signs of degeneration and disintegration (karyorrhexis, karyolysis). Hematoxylin and eosin (×360).

were as follows: 0, less than 6 neutrophils; 1, 6–40 neutrophils; 2, more than 40 neutrophils with moderate numbers of focal collections and/or relatively few scattered neutrophils; 3, more than 40 neutrophils with extensive foci and relatively few neutrophils scattered, or relatively few foci and moderate numbers scattered; 4, extensive foci and marked numbers of neutrophils scattered. The scores obtained for the two areas were then added to provide a total score for the section (possible range 0–8).

B. Local Application

Intradermal injection in the rat of 10^{-9} mol of IL-8 or PAF induced emigration of neutrophils from small vessels as early as 10 min after application, whereas 10^{-13} mol of endotoxin had no effect (Fig. 1). Within 30 min after IL-8 application there was a distinct intraluminar, vessel wall, and perivascular accumulation of neutrophils, especially in and around venules in the lower dermis (Fig. 2a). A striking finding was the presence of massive neutrophil aggregates between the endothelial and smooth muscle layers of the vessel wall. At the same time point, PAF caused a milder and more diffuse perivascular accumulation of neutrophils, whereas endotoxin and PFS did not cause any significant inflammatory reaction (Figs. 1 and 3). One hour after application of IL-8 there was still a high number of neutrophils in the vessel walls (Fig. 2b) and an increasing number in perivascular spaces. The intensity of the neutrophilic infiltrate was much more pronounced after injection of IL-8 than after injection of PAF or endotoxin. Neutrophil infiltration peaked at 4 hr after injection of IL-8 and PAF. Similar to the 1-hr time point, at 4 hr the infiltration score of IL-8 sites was distinctly higher than the scores for PAF or endotoxin sites. At this time point, IL-8 caused a massive neutrophilic infiltration of the upper and lower dermis with areas of diffuse distribution of neutrophils (Fig. 2c) and areas with dense, microabscess-like neutrophil accumulation, mainly around venules in the deep dermis. Focally the inflammatory infiltrate extended into the panniculus carnosus. After 8 hr and especially after 16 hr a decrease in the number of neutrophils in the inflammatory infiltrate could be observed, except for the endotoxin-treated sites, where the number remained comparable to the 4-hr value. The neutrophils in the IL-8-treated sites demonstrated signs of degeneration such as cell swelling, pycnosis, karyorrhexis, and karyolysis (Fig. 2d). The inflammatory score of IL-8-treated sites decreased steadily over the next 12 hr, and was back to the levels of the untreated sites at the end of the observation period (Fig. 3).

We also compared the activity of different doses of IL-8,. NAP-2, and GRO-α 4 hr after intradermal injection into rats. All three substances induced a dose-dependent accumulation of neutrophils. However, the magnitude of the inflammatory reaction was different with the three inflammatory pep-

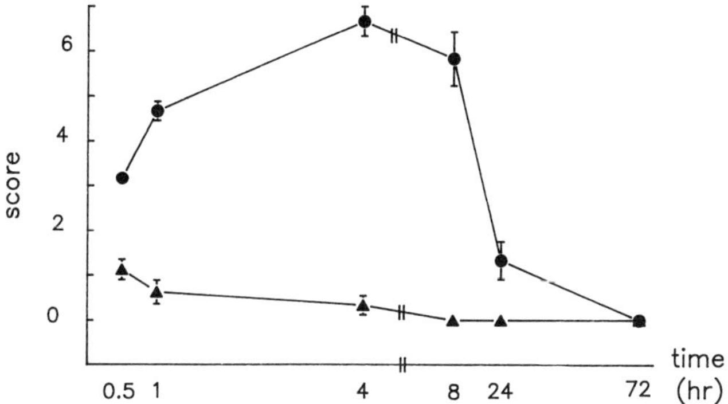

Fig. 3. Inflammatory score after a single intradermal injection of IL-8 or PFS in rats. Comparison between values ± SEM for PFS-injected sites (▲, n = 4–8) and values ± SEM for sites injected with 10^{-9} mol of IL-8 (●, n = 8).

tides tested. GRO-α induced an appreciable intradermal neutrophil accumulation at 10^{-11} mol/site, whereas at 10^{-10} and especially 10^{-9} mol/site it caused an extremely strong inflammatory reaction (Figs. 4b and 5). IL-8 induced a slightly weaker but still substantial inflammatory reaction (Fig. 5), whereas NAP-2 elicited a much lower number of neutrophils than the other two agonists (Fig. 5).

C. Systemic Application

A single i.v. IL-8 injection induced a marked neutrophilia in Chinchilla rabbits, which was present after 15 min and peaked between 1 and 2 hr and remained marked until the end of the observation period (Table II). Histological examination revealed leukostasis and congestion in dilated lung vessels of IL-8-treated animals (not shown). Repeated short-term IL-8 injections induced significant histological changes only in the lung. Neutrophil aggregates were found in small to medium-sized lung vessels, whereas accumulation of individual neutrophils could be observed in lung capillaries. Additionally, diffuse septal edema and foci of hemorrhage and intraalveolar edema were observed (Fig. 6a). Animals that had received five daily IL-8 injections showed a substantial broadening of the alveolar septa, which contained a large number of fibroblasts, type II pneumocytes, and a mixed inflammatory cellular infiltrate consisting of small and large mononuclear cells and neutrophils (Fig. 6b). Focal atelectasis and alveoli with homogeneous eosinophilic exudate were also present. After a recovery period of 2 weeks, major areas of the lung tissue were histologically normal; however, some extended areas consisted of large distorted alveoli with expanded air

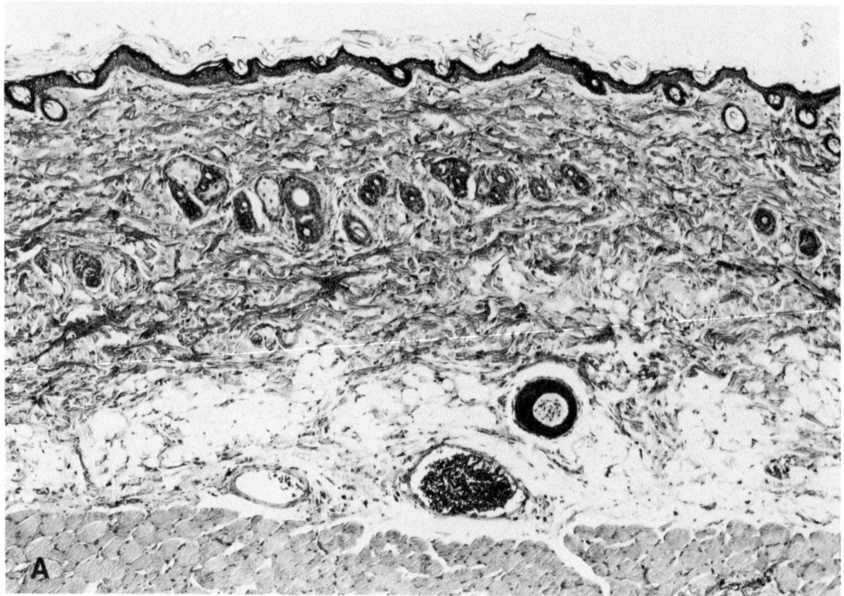

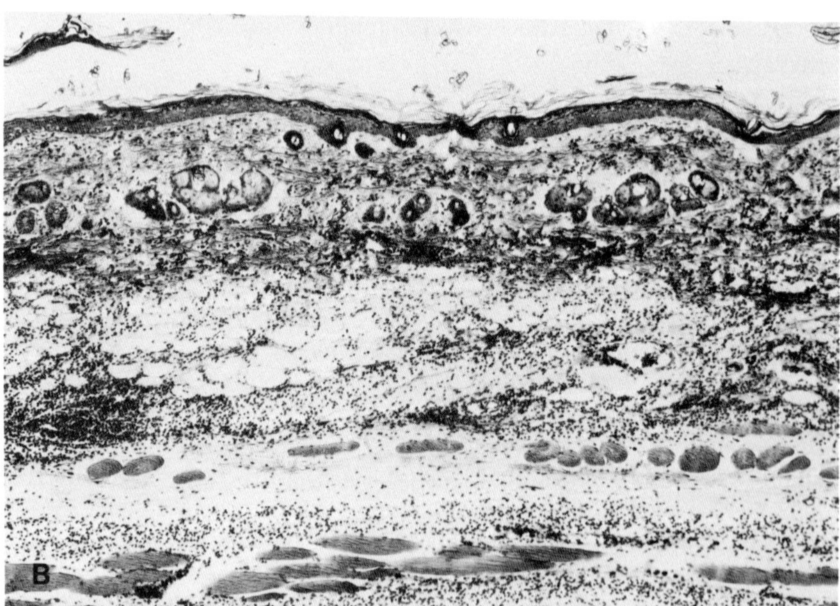

Fig. 4. Rat skin 4 hours after intradermal injection of (a) PFS or (b) 10^{-9} mol of GRO-α. (a) Slight edema of lower dermis, no change in vessels. (b) Massive and extensive neutrophil infiltration of all dermal layers with formation of microabscess-like foci in perivenular areas. Hematoxylin and eosin ($\times$50).

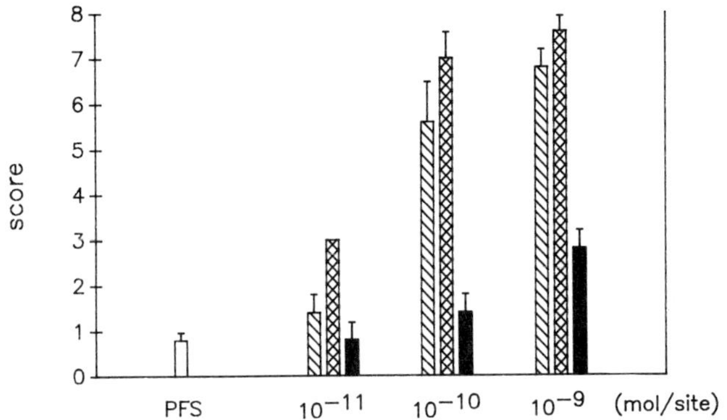

Fig. 5. Inflammatory score 4 hr after a single intradermal injection of different agonists in rats. Comparison between values ± SEM of sites injected with PFS (open bar), IL-8 (hatched bars), GRO-α (cross-hatched bars), and NAP-2 (filled bars).

spaces, and showed signs of destruction of the alveolar septa closely resembling those seen in human emphysema. Other reactive patterns were represented by lung areas with wide alveoli lined by type II pneumocytes and alveolar septa thickened by mononuclear cells, neutrophils, and fibroblasts, and the presence of collagen deposition.

V. DISCUSSION

Injection of human IL-8 into rat skin induced a rapid and concentration-dependent neutrophil infiltration. Within 30–60 min after injection of IL-8, neutrophils accumulated within the vessel wall and moderate numbers of

Table II. Relative Hematology Values of Two Rabbits[a]

Time after injection	Lymphocytes		Neutrophils		Monocytes	
	A	B	A	B	A	B
0 min	1.00	1.00	1.00	1.00	1.00	1.00
15 min	1.24	1.56	3.49	1.74	3.32	0.52
30 min	1.53	2.03	6.79	28.7	0	2.87
1 hr	1.49	1.62	4.55	45.5	0.41	1.12
2 hr	0.67	0.89	7.3	37.6	0	0
4 hr	0.85	1.34	5.69	35.1	1.42	0
7 hr	0.91	1.31	3.25	15.6	0.54	0

[a] Rabbits (A and B) were injected with a single i.v. bolus of 100 μg (11.9 nmol) of IL-8.

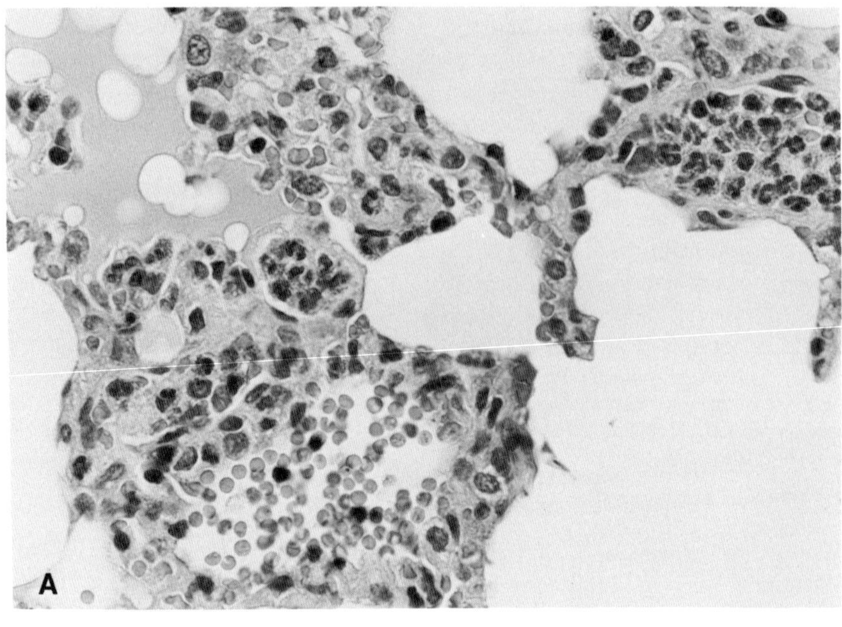

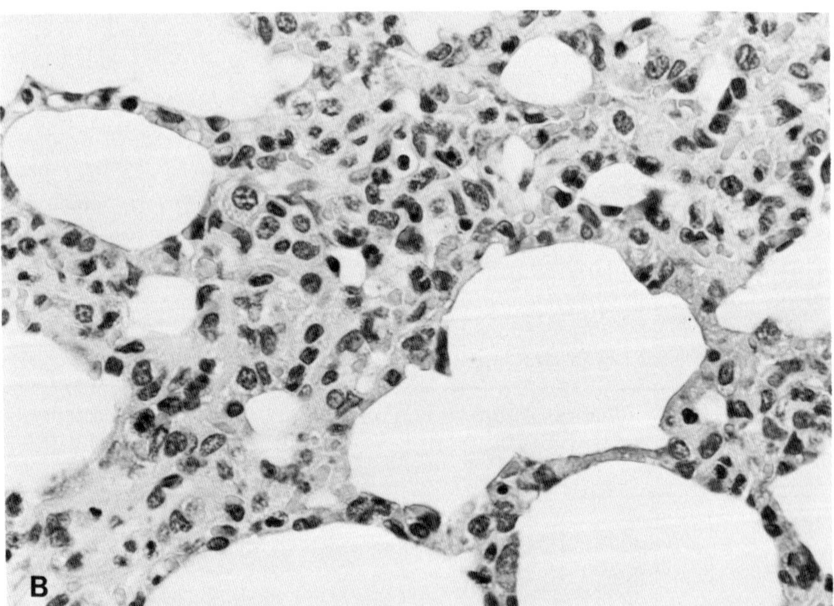

Fig. 6. Rabbit lungs after intravenous injection of IL-8. (a) At 2 hr after three i.v. injections of 100 μg (12 nmol) of IL-8. Note intravascular accumulation of neutrophils, congestion, and focal intraalveolar edema (top). (b) At 2 hr after five daily i.v. injections of 5 nmol of IL-8. Note interstitial mixed inflammatory infiltrate with fibroblast proliferation. Hematoxylin and eosin.

cells were already present in the perivascular tissue. The observed formation of subendothelial neutrophil aggregates was unusual and has not been observed for other chemotactic agonists, such as C5a, PAF, or endotoxin. After injection of IL-8, neutrophil infiltration was more intense than is observed for PAF and endotoxin. Interestingly, neutrophils in the perivascular space disappeared after 16 to 24 hr, leaving no signs of tissue damage, indicating that neutrophil activation had not occurred and that proteolytic enzymes were not released from the disintegrating neutrophils.

In vivo mobilization of neutrophils induced by IL-8 in intradermal sites has been previously described in rats (Larsen *et al.,* 1989; Rot, 1991), rabbits (Colditz *et al.,* 1989; Foster *et al.,* 1989; Rampart *et al.,* 1989; Rot, 1991), dogs (Thomsen *et al.,* 1991), and man (Leonard *et al.,* 1991a; Swensson *et al.,* 1991). In agreement with our results obtained in rat skin, no lymphocyte or basophil infiltration, nor evidence for mast cell degranulation, was observed after IL-8 injection in the human, rabbit, and dog. However, lymphocyte emigration induced by very low concentrations of human IL-8 in the rat has been described (Larsen *et al.,* 1989; Rot, 1991). In the human studies, Leonard *et al.* did not observe a significant percentage of monocyte accumulation in perivascular areas, whereas Swensson *et al.* did. This monocyte infiltration could possibly be caused by the release of monocyte chemoattractants, such as CAP37, from emigrated neutrophils (Pereira *et al.,* 1989).

In the rat skin, both IL-8 and GRO-α induced a similar and dose-dependent neutrophil infiltration, whereas NAP-2 was significantly less potent. However, in the rabbit skin, IL-8 and NAP-2 were of identical potency (Walz *et al.,* 1991b). The reason for this interspecies difference is not clear, but the *in vivo* results correlate with the relative *in vitro* chemotactic potencies of IL-8 and NAP-2 for rat neutrophils (A. Rot, unpublished observations). Species-specific differences in the structure of receptors for those inflammatory peptides could account for this discrepancy.

The repeated systemic application of human IL-8 in rabbits caused neutrophil sequestration in the lung and signs of increased vascular permeability, followed by development of inflammatory and proliferative changes in lung interstitium. The lesions observed in lung vessels and tissues could be explained by local neutrophil activation, which in turn could lead to tissue damage and increased vascular permeability (Till *et al.,* 1982). The proliferative changes observed are probably secondary to the tissue damage and the release of additional mediators, such as platelet-derived growth factor (Snyder *et al.,* 1991).

The fact that proinflammatory cytokines such as IL-1 and TNF induce the synthesis of IL-8 in many different cell types suggests its involvement in a wide range of physiologic and pathologic conditions. High levels of IL-8 and IL-1 were found in scales of patients with psoriasis (Sticherling *et al.,* 1991) and in synovial fluid of patients with rheumatoid arthritis (Seitz *et al.,* 1991).

Enhanced chemotactic activity for neutrophils has also been observed in the bronchoalveolar lavage fluid of patients with adult respiratory distress syndrome (Parsons *et al.,* 1985), idiopathic pulmonary fibrosis (Hunninghake *et al.,* 1981), and asbestosis (Hayes *et al.,* 1988). The demonstration of the *in vivo* activity of IL-8 and related neutrophil-activating peptides in man and animals strongly suggests their important role in the pathophysiology of inflammatory diseases.

VI. SUMMARY

Interleukin-8 is a member of a novel cytokine family and has been found to be an activator and attractant for human neutrophils *in vitro.* The *in vivo* activity was tested in experimental animal models by intradermal and intravenous administration of IL-8. Intradermal administration of human IL-8 in rats induces a rapid and concentration-dependent neutrophil infiltration, which peaks 4 hr after IL-8 application. Injection of GRO-α induces a similar chemotactic response, whereas neutrophil-activating peptide-2 was significantly less active. When injected intravenously into rabbits, IL-8 induced neutrophil sequestration in the lungs and, following repeated injections, caused septal and intraalveolar edema and lung damage resembling that seen in adult respiratory distress syndrome. The fact that IL-8 is induced and secreted from many different cell types suggests its involvement in a variey of physiologic and pathologic conditions as a neutrophil chemoattractant and, possibly, as an activator of other neutrophil responses.

References

Anisowicz, A., Bardwell, L., and Sager, R. (1987). *Proc. Natl. Acad. Sci. U.S.A.* **84,** 7188.

Bacon, K. B., Westwick, J., and Camp, R. D. (1989). *Biochem. Biophys. Res. Commun.* **165,** 349.

Baggiolini, M., Dewald, B., and Walz, A. *In* "Inflammation: Basic Principles and Clinical Correlates" (J. I. Gallin, I. M. Goldstein, and R. Snyderman, eds.) (in press). Raven, New York.

Car, B. D., Baggiolini, M., and Walz, A. (1991). *Biochem. J.* **275,** 581.

Carveth, H. J., Bohnsack, J. F., McIntyre, T. M., Baggiolini, M., Prescott, S. M., and Zimmerman, G. A. (1989). *Biochem. Biophys. Res. Commun.* **162,** 387.

Colditz, I., Zwahlen, R., Dewald, B., and Baggiolini, M. (1989). *Am. J. Pathol.* **134,** 755.

Dahinden, C. A., Kurimoto, Y., De Weck, A. L., Lindley, I., Dewald, B., and Baggiolini, M. (1989). *J. Exp. Med.* **170,** 1787.

Detmers, P. A., Lo, S. K., Olsen-Egbert, E., Walz, A., Baggiolini, M., and Cohn, Z. A. (1990). *J. Exp. Med.* **171,** 1155.

Fernandez, H. N., Henson, P. M., Otani, A., and Hugli, T. E. (1978). *J. Immunol.* **120,** 109.

Ford Hutchinson, A. W., Bray, M. A., Doig, M. V., Shipley, M. E., and Smith, M. J. (1980). *Nature (London)* **286,** 264.

Foster, A., Aked, D. M., Schroeder, J.-M., and Christophers, E. (1989). *Immunology* **67,** 181.

Haskill, S., Peace, A., Morris, J., Sporn, S. A., Anisowicz, A., Lee, S. W., Smith, T., Martin, G., Ralph, P., and Sager, R. (1990). *Proc. Natl. Acad. Sci. U.S.A.* **87**, 7732.

Hayes, A. A., Rose, A. H., Musk, A. W., and Robinson, B. W. (1988). *Chest* **94**, 521.

Hunninghake, G. W., Gadek, J. E., Lawley, T. J., and Crystal, R. G. (1981). *J. Clin. Invest.* **68**, 259.

Larsen, C. G., Anderson, A. O., Appella, E., Oppenheim, J. J., and Matsushima, K. (1989). *Science* **243**, 1464.

Leonard, E. J., Skeel, A., Yoshimura, T., Noer, K., Kutvirt, S., and Van Epps, D. (1990). *J. Immunol.* **144**, 1323.

Leonard, E. J., Yoshimura, T., Tanaka, S., and Raffeld, M. (1991a). *J. Invest. Dermatol.* **96**, 690.

Leonard, E. J., Yoshimura, T., Rot, A., Noer, K., Walz, A., Baggiolini, M., Walz, D. A., Goetz, E. J., and Castor, C. W. (1991b). *J. Leukocyte Biol.* **49**, 258.

Lindley, I., Aschauer, H., Seifert, J. M., Lam, C., Brunowsky, W., Kownatzki, E., Thelen, M., Peveri, P., Dewald, B., von Tscharner, V., Walz, A., and Baggiolini, M. (1988). *Proc. Natl. Acad. Sci. U.S.A.* **85**, 9199.

Moser, B., Clark-Lewis, I., Zwahlen, R., and Baggiolini, M. (1990) *J. Exp. Med.* **171**, 1797.

Munro, J. M., Pober, J. S., and Cotran, R. S. (1989). *Am. J. Pathol.* **135**, 121.

Oppenheim, J. J., Zachariae, C. O. C., Mukaida, N., and Matsushima, K. (1991). *Annu. Rev. Immunol.* **9**, 617.

Paccaud, J.-P., Schifferli, J. A., and Baggiolini, M. (1990). *Biochem. Biophys. Res. Commun.* **166**, 187.

Parsons, P. E., Fowler, A. A., Hyers, T. M., and Henson, P. M. (1985). *Am. Rev. Respir. Dis.* **132**, 490.

Pereira, H. A., Shafer, W. M., Pohl, J., Martin, L. E., and Spitznagel, J. K. (1989). *J. Clin. Invest.* **85**, 1468.

Rampart, M., Van Damme, J., Honnekeyn, L., and Herman, A. G. (1989). *Am. J. Pathol.* **135**, 21.

Richmond, A., and Thomas, H. G. (1988). *J. Cell. Biochem.* **36**, 185.

Rot, A. (1991). *Cytokine* **3**, 21.

Rot, A., Henderson, L. E., Copeland, T. D., and Leonard, E. J. (1987). *Proc. Natl. Acad. Sci. U.S.A.* **84**, 7967.

Schall, T. J. (1991). *Cytokine* **3**, 165.

Schiffmann, E., Corcoran, B. A., and Wahl, S. M. (1975). *Proc. Natl. Acad. Sci. U.S.A.* **72**, 1059.

Schroeder, J. M., Mrowietz, U., Morita, E., and Christophers, E. (1987). *J. Immunol.* **139**, 3474.

Seitz, M., Dewald, B., Gerber, N., and Baggiolini, M. (1991). *J. Clin. Invest.* **87**, 463.

Shaw, J. O., Pinckard, R. N., Ferrigni, K. S., McManus, L. M., and Hanahan, D. J. (1981). *J. Immunol.* **127**, 1250.

Snyder, L. S., Hertz, M. I., Peterson, M. S., Harmon, K. R., Marinelli, W. A., Henke, C. A., Greenheck, J. R., Chen, B., and Bitterman, P. B. (1991). *J. Clin. Invest.* **88**, 663.

Sticherling, M., Bornscheuer, E., Schroeder, J.-M., and Christophers, E. (1991). *J. Invest. Dermatol.* **96**, 26.

Swensson, O., Schubert, C., Christophers, E., and Schroeder, J.-M. (1991). *J. Invest. Dermatol.* **96**, 682.

Tekamp-Olson, P., Gallegos, C., Bauer, D., McClain, J., Sherry, B., Fabre, M., Van Deventer, S., and Cerami, A. (1990). *J. Exp. Med.* **172**, 911.

Thomsen, M. K., Larsen, C. G., Thomsen, H. K., Kirstein, D., Skak-Nielsen, T., Ahnfelt-Ronne, I., and Thestrup-Pederson, K. (1991). *J. Invest. Dermatol.* **96**, 260.

Till, G. O., Johnson, K. J., Kunkel, R., and Ward, P. A. (1982). *J. Clin. Invest.* **69**, 1126.

Walz, A. (1991). *In* "Cytokines; Neutrophil-Activating Peptides and Other Chemotactic Cytokines" Vol. 4, pp. 77–95 (C. Sorg and M. Baggiolini, eds.). Karger, Basel.

Walz, A., and Baggiolini, M. (1989). *Biochem. Biophys. Res. Commun.* **159**, 969.

Walz, A., and Baggiolini, M. (1990). *J. Exp. Med.* **171**, 449.

Walz, A., Peveri, P., Aschauer, H., and Baggiolini, M. (1987). *Biochem. Biophys. Res. Commun.*

149, 755.

Walz, A., Dewald, B., von Tscharner, V., and Baggiolini, M. (1989). *J. Exp. Med.* **170,** 1745.

Walz, A., Meloni, F., Clark-Lewis, I.,von Tscharner, V., and Baggiolini, M. (1991a). *J. Leukocyte Biol.* **50,** 279.

Walz, A., Zwahlen, R., and Baggiolini, M. (1991b). *Adv. Exp. Med. Biol.* **305,** 39.

Waringa, R. A. J., Koenderman, L., Kok, P. T. M., Kreukniet, J., and Bruijnzeel, P. L. B. (1991). *Blood* **77,** 2694.

Yoshimura, T., Matsushima, K., Oppenheim, J. J., and Leonard, E. J. (1987). *J. Immunol.* **139,** 788.

Pathology of Recombinant Human Transforming Growth Factor-β1 in Rats and Rabbits

Timothy G. Terrell
Department of Safety Evaluation
Genentech, Inc.
South San Francisco, California 94080

Peter K. Working
Department of Pharmacology and Toxicology
Liposome Technologies, Inc.
Menlo Park, California 94025

C. Paul Chow and James D. Green
Department of Safety Evaluation
Genentech, Inc.,
South San Francisco, California 94080

I. INTRODUCTION

Transforming growth factor-$\beta1$ (TGF-$\beta1$) was originally described as a peptide that caused reversible transformation of rodent fibroblasts (Moses *et al.,* 1981; Roberts *et al.,* 1981). The assay used to measure this activity, which provided the name for the peptide, was the ability of TGF-$\beta1$ to induce normal rat kidney fibroblasts to grow and form colonies in soft agar in the presence of epidermal growth factor (De Larco and Todaro, 1978). TGF-$\beta1$ also stimulates anchorage-independent growth of other fibroblastic cell lines (Moses *et al.,* 1981; Massagué *et al.,* 1985). TGF-$\beta1$ was first purified to homogeneity from human platelets (Assoian *et al.,* 1983) and was characterized as a dimeric peptide composed of two identical 112-amino acid subunits with a molecular mass of 25,000 Da. The cloning of human TGF-β1 and the resulting elucidation of its precursor structure (Derynck *et al.,* 1985) have led to identification of five other forms of TGF-β (Massagué, 1990). TGF-β1 is the structural prototype of a family of structurally and functionally related factors involved in growth, differentiation, and morphogenesis (Massagué, 1987). The individual TGF-βs are extremely well conserved across species. There is greater than 99% identity between the mature TGF-β1 sequences of various mammalian species (Derynck *et al.,* 1986, 1987).

Numerous cell types have been shown to produce or express one or more forms of TGF-β, and expression of TGF-β1 is active throughout embryonic development and into adulthood (Heine *et al.,* 1987). Localization of TGF-β1 or its mRNA by immunohistochemistry or *in situ* hybridization has shown that it is expressed in many embryonic tissues with characteristic temporal patterns (Lehnert and Akhurst, 1988; Wilcox and Derynck, 1988), suggesting that it plays an important role in normal development. TGF-β is secreted from cells in a biologically inactive form, which lacks the ability to bind to the TGF-β receptor (Wakefield *et al.,* 1987). The exact mechanism of activation of latent TGF-β1 *in vivo* is not known, but may involve proteases or exposure to acid microenvironments. Because the cellular receptor for TGF-β1 appears to be universally expressed, the target specificity of TGF-β1 action may be determined by the ability of cells to activate the latent form of the molecule (Sporn and Roberts, 1987). Once activated, TGF-β1 is very rapidly cleared from the circulation by a process that apparently involves binding to α_2-macroglobulin (LaMarre *et al.,* 1991).

The range of cell types that respond to TGF-β1 and the variety of cellular responses elicited by the molecule are diverse (Table I). The name for the factor, transforming growth factor, is misleading, because it does not cause oncogenic transformation and is actually one of the most potent growth inhibitors known. TGF-β1 has reversible growth inhibitory activity on epithelial, endothelial, fibroblastic, neuronal, lymphoid, and hematopoietic cells *in vitro* (Massagué, 1990), and this inhibitory effect has also been demonstrated *in vivo* (Russell *et al.,* 1988; Silberstein and Daniel, 1987). Some mesenchymal cells proliferate in response to TGF-β1, although this response may not represent a direct effect of the cytokine, but may be secondary to production of autocrine mitogens (Massagué, 1987). TGF-βs inhibit adipogenesis, myogenesis, and hematopoiesis, whereas they promote chondrogenesis and epithelial cell differentiation. TGF-β1 is a potent stimulator of extracellular matrix production by fibroblasts and osteoblasts (Sporn *et al.,* 1987). This is accomplished through increased synthesis of matrix proteins and inhibitors of proteases, and decreased production of proteases (Moses, 1990). TGF-β1 is also one of the most potent chemotactic agents for macrophages that has been identified (Wahl *et al.,* 1987). The net effect of these

Table I. Biological Activities of TGF-β[a]

Cell proliferation
Inhibition: Epithelium, endothelium, fibroblasts,
lymphocytes, hematopoietic cells
Stimulation: Fibroblasts, osteoblasts

Cell differentiation
Inhibition: Preadipocytes, myoblasts, megakaryocytes,
hematopoietic progenitor cells, lymphocytes
Stimulation: Prechrondroblasts, osteoblasts, epithelium,
keratinocytes

Accumulation of extracellular matrix
Stimulation of extracellular matrix synthesis
Inhibition of extracellular matrix degradation
Up-regulates protease inhibitors
Down-regulates proteolytic enzymes

Increases cell adhesion
Stimulates synthesis of integrin receptors
Stimulates integrin synthesis

Chemotaxis
Macrophages
Fibroblasts
Osteoblasts

---

[a] From Massagué (1990) and Roberts and Sporn (1990).

properties *in vivo* include stimulation of granulation tissue formation
(Roberts *et al.,* 1986), promotion of wound healing (Mustoe *et al.,* 1987;
Beck *et al.,* 1990), and immunosuppression (Wallick *et al.,* 1990). The many
functions and widespread expression of TGF-β1 and its receptor suggest that
it plays an important role in many physiological and pathological processes.
Experiments in several animal models have demonstrated that recombinant human transforming growth factor-β1 (rHuTGF-β1) can promote
wound healing when applied topically. In addition to its effect on increasing
the strength of incisional wounds, it has been shown to accelerate healing of
an open wound (Ammann *et al.,* 1990). Based on this demonstrated activity,
rHuTGF-β1 was evaluated for its potential clinical use as a wound-healing
agent. A series of preclinical safety studies were conducted in rats and rabbits
(Table II). In dermal studies, rHuTGF-β1 was applied to open wounds under
conditions designed to mimic the clinical use of the compound. In addition,
intravenous toxicity studies were conducted to evaluate the effects of systemic exposure to rHuTGF-β1. With the exception of one pilot study in
which rHuTGF-β expressed in a human embryonic kidney cell line (A293)

Table II. Nonclinical Toxicology Studies with rHuTGF-β1

Acute toxicology
    Rat
        Intravenous
        Dermal
    Rabbit
        Intravenous
        Dermal

Pilot multidose study (A293 cell material)
    Rat
        Intravenous, 14 days

Subchronic toxicology
    Rat
        Intravenous, 4 weeks
        Dermal, 4 weeks
    Rabbit
        Dermal, 4 weeks

was used, all studies were conducted with rHuTGF-β1 expressed in Chinese hamster ovarian (CHO) cells.

II. EXPERIMENTAL RESULTS

A. Dermal Toxicity Studies

Acute single-dose dermal toxicity studies were conducted in rats and rabbits using a formulation containing 1.0 mg/ml in 3% methylcellulose gel. In rats, the gel was applied to two wound sites, which were created using an 8 mm diameter Baker/Cumins biopsy punch, and in rabbits it was applied to a 2 cm × 2 cm surgical wound. In both species, the dose applied was 200 μg/cm^2 of wound site, which is approximately 80 times the dose shown to be efficacious in promoting wound healing (Beck *et al.*, 1990). Rats were necropsied 1, 3, 6, and 15 days after treatment. Gross and microscopic examination of the wound sites showed no differences between the rHuTGF-β1-treated and control animals, and normal healing profiles were observed in both groups.

Rabbits were examined 2 weeks after treatment. Histopathological change at the treatment site of rHuTGF-β1-treated rabbits included reduced re-epithelialization (Fig. 1) with failure of the epidermis to proliferate and migrate over the surface of the wound (Fig. 2). All control animals had an

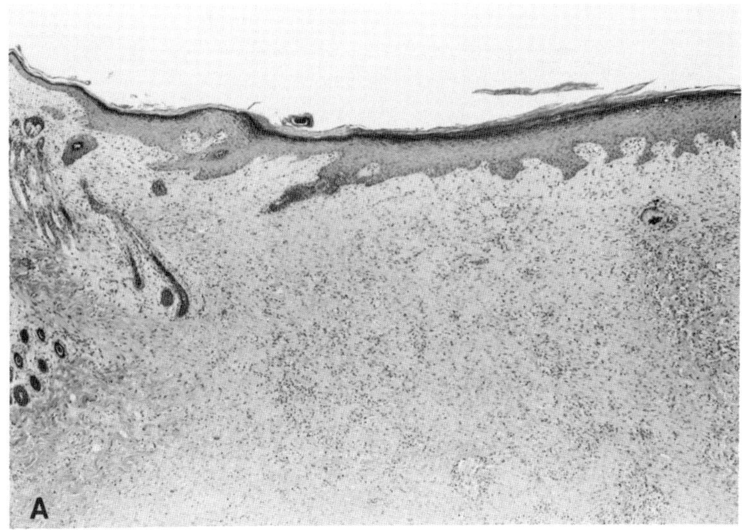

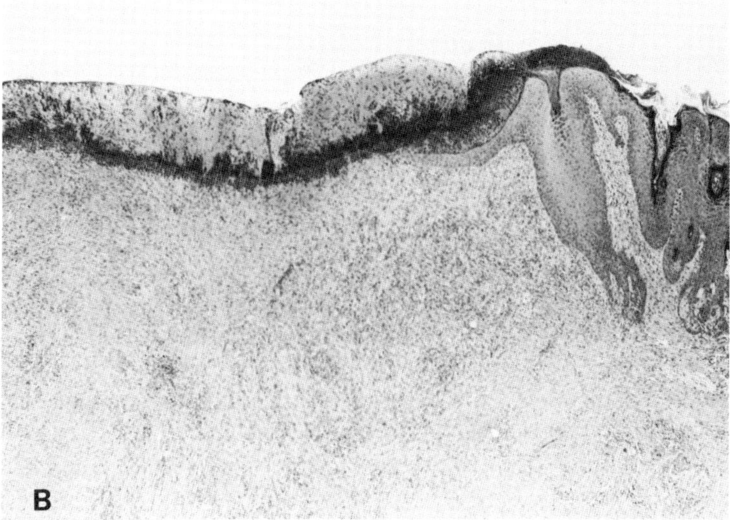

Fig. 1. Skin from wound site of rabbits 2 weeks after the wound was created. (a) Control rabbit treated with excipient gel showing intact epithelial surface overlying area of proliferation of granulation tissue. Hematoxylin and eosin (×40). (b) Rabbit treated with rHuTGF-β1 gel formulation (200 μg/cm²). There is a failure of the epithelium to proliferate over the wound site, with increased proliferation of granulation tissue and inflammatory cell infiltration. Hematoxylin and eosin (×40).

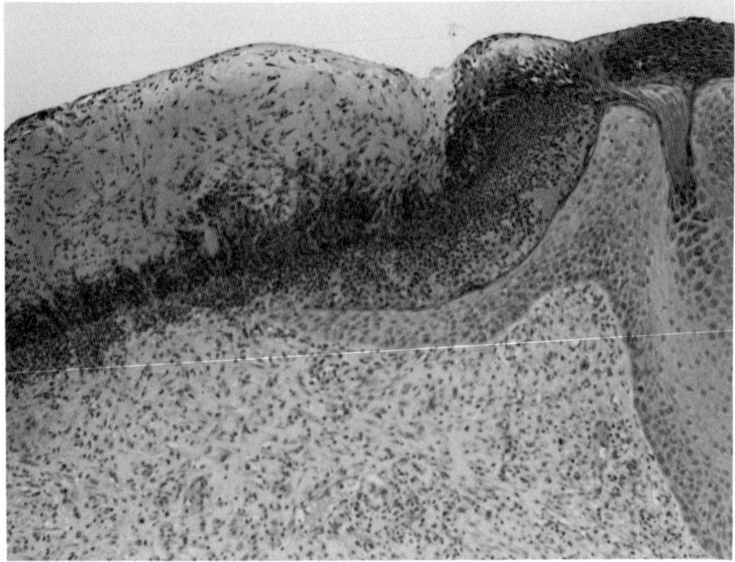

Fig. 2. Higher magnification of the lesion in Fig. 1 showing the leading edge of the proliferating surface epithelium. Hematoxylin and eosin (×100).

intact epidermal covering of the wound sites. Other microscopic changes included an increase in the amount of granulation tissue formation, increased leukocytic infiltration, and the presence of a superficial exudate of proteinaceous material and neutrophils on the open wound.

In a subacute dermal study, rHuTGF-β1 was applied topically to wound sites in rats for 31 consecutive days with doses up to 90 μg/cm^2. Wound sites were created with a 6 mm diameter Baker/Cumins biopsy punch and were full-thickness wounds of the skin extending to the underlying muscle layer. The rHuTGF-β1 gel was applied daily as a 50-μl aliquot for a 6-hr exposure period at doses of 0.05, 1.25, or 25 μg per animal (up to 90 μg/cm^2 wound site). Each wound site was treated for consecutively for 7 days, and new wounds were created at 7-day intervals throughout the 4-week study. Five rats of each sex were maintained for an additional 4-week treatment-free recovery period after cessation of treatment. In addition to daily observations for clinical signs of systemic toxicity, parameters evaluated at the end of the treatment and recovery periods included ophthalmic examinations, clinical pathology evaluations, analysis for antibody formation, gross pathology, organ weights, and microscopic examination of a comprehensive set of tissues.

There were no overt signs of toxicity in any of the clinical parameters evaluated or in hematology serum chemistry or urinalysis parameters. No antibody formation to rHuTGF-β1 was observed in treated animals. No gross lesions were observed in the treated animals and organ weights were comparable to control animals. Histopathological changes at the wound sites of both control and treated animals were characteristic of changes associated with normal wound healing. The study design permitted histopathological characterization of the wound sites at weekly intervals from 1 to 8 weeks duration (wounds created on study days 21, 14, 7, and 0; terminal and recovery sacrifices, respectively). There was morphological variation between wound sites on individual animals, which reflected the chronological progression of the healing process. Reepithelialization of the wound site was completed by the first interval evaluated, 7 days. The epithelium was moderately acanthotic with hyperkeratosis. The open wound was completely filled in with actively proliferating granulation tissue and mild, mixed inflammatory cell infiltrates. The epidermal changes (acanthosis and hyperkeratosis) had resolved by 3 weeks. Dermal changes showed a progressive decrease in active proliferation, or fibroplasia, and inflammatory cell infiltration of the wound, with increasing deposition of collagen from weeks 1–3. There was then a progressive condensation and organization of the collagen deposits, leading to formation of a normal scar by the end of the recovery period. This scar was composed of dense collagen in the dermis, was devoid of adnexal structures, and was covered by normal epidermis. No histopathological differences were observed between treated and control animals.

A comparable dermal toxicity study was conducted in rabbits in which the rHuTGF-β1 gel was topically applied to surgical wounds of 3 cm^2 at doses of 5, 15, and 40 μg/cm^2. The same parameters were evaluated as in the 4-week rat study, except that blood for hematology and serum chemistry evaluation was collected after 1 and 2 weeks of treatment in addition to the terminal and recovery sacrifice intervals. In this study there was no evidence of systemic toxicity, and no histopathological difference was noted between wound sites of treated and control animals.

B. Intravenous Toxicity Studies

Acute intravenous toxicity studies were conducted in rats and rabbits with rHuTGF-β1 at doses of 100, 300, and 860 μg/kg body weight. Animals were administered a single intravenous bolus injection into the lateral tail vein (rats) or marginal ear vein (rabbits) at a dose volume of 1.0 ml/kg; a 2-week observation period followed. Animals were observed for clinical signs of toxicity. Blood for clinical pathology parameters was collected on day 3 (rabbit only), day 5 (rats only), and at the end of the observation period. All animals received a complete necropsy examination, and injection veins from the rabbits were examined microscopically.

There were no clinical signs of overt toxicity nor any treatment-related gross lesions in the rats. A mild, reversible thrombocytopenia was observed at all doses of rHuTGF-β1 tested.

Rabbits treated with midlevel or high doses of rHuTGF-β1 had a transient reduction in food consumption and weight loss. Males receiving the high dose had slightly lower albumin, total protein, urea nitrogen, and calcium levels on day 3; however, these changes were essentially reversed by 2 weeks. There were no systemic gross pathology changes; however, local tissue reactions were present around the injection vein, with nodular thickening or firmness of the pinna. Histopathologically, the change was characterized by increased amounts of fibrotic connective tissue formation in the perivascular adventitial tissue. This fibrosis was attributed to a response to extravenous deposition or leakage of the test formulation during administration.

Two multidose intravenous studies were conducted with rHuTGF-β1. Initially, a pilot 14-day range-finding study using an early formulation of rHuTGF-β1 expressed in the human cell line A293 was performed. Rats were administered intravenous bolus injections of rHuTGF-β1 at doses of 10, 100, and 1000 μg/kg for 14 consecutive days. Blood was collected under ketamine anesthesia on days 3, 6, 9, and at termination of treatment for hematology and serum chemistry parameters. Because of deaths in two high-dose males after 5 treatments, all surviving high-dose animals were euthanized on day 6. All other animals survived until the scheduled termination of the study after 14 days. A complete necropsy examination was performed on all animals, and selected organs were weighed and/or examined histologically.

Adverse effects attributed to rHuTGF-β1 were most striking in the high-dose group (1000 μg/kg/day), which were sacrificed after 5 days of treatment. Qualitatively similar changes were observed at the mid-dose level; however, they were generally much less severe and delayed in onset. Body weights were decreased in high-dose animals as early as study day 3. Mid-dose group animals exhibited a decrease in body weight gain, which was evident at 6 days of dosing through the end of the treatment period. Animals in the mid- and high-dose groups had increased hematocrits compared to controls on day 3, suggesting a degree of hemoconcentration. Subsequently, a progressive decrease in values for hematocrit and hemoglobin was observed in all rHuTGF-β1-treated groups during the treatment period, and values were significantly lower than controls on day 15 (Fig. 3). High-dose animals showed marked increases in serum alkaline phosphatase (ALP), aspartate aminotransferase (AST), total bilirubin, and cholesterol, and decreases in glucose, phosphorus, albumin, and total protein (Fig. 4). These changes were evident at day 3 and increased in magnitude by day 6. Mid-dose groups also had increased ALP, AST, and cholesterol, and a slight

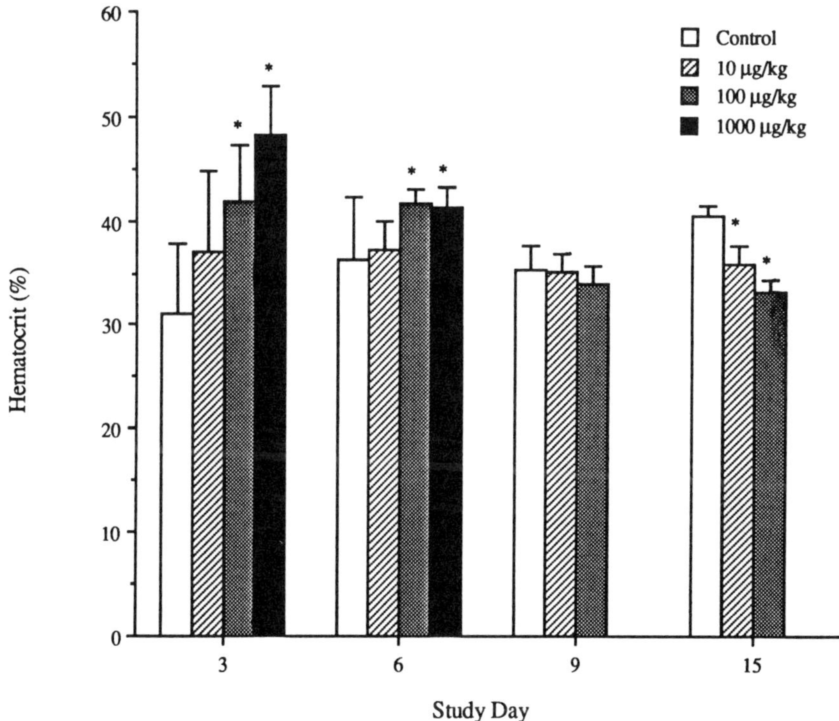

Study Day

Fig. 3. Mean hematocrits for rats treated intravenously with rHuTGF-β1 for 14 days. Data for male animals only are shown, but similar results were present in females. High-dose animals were sacrificed after 5 days of treatment. Statistically significant differences when compared to controls of same sex using the Student's *t* test are indicated (*, $p < 0.05$).

decrease in albumin. No changes in serum chemistry values were observed for low-dose animals.

A very dramatic decrease in liver weight (to approximately 30% of control group values) was observed in the high-dose group (Fig. 5). This hepatic involution occurred after only 5 days of treatment. Liver weights were also decreased in the mid-dose group, and heart and spleen weights were decreased in mid- and high-dose groups.

Histopathological changes attributed to effects of the rHuTGF-β1 were observed in multiple organs and tissues, including liver, kidney, heart, thymus, bone, pancreas, stomach, cecum, at the injection vein, and in skeletal muscle at the site of anesthetic (ketamine hydrochloride) injection (Table III). Lesions were observed primarily in animals treated with 100 or 1000 μg/kg/day of rHuTGF-β1, with a dose-related increase in incidence and

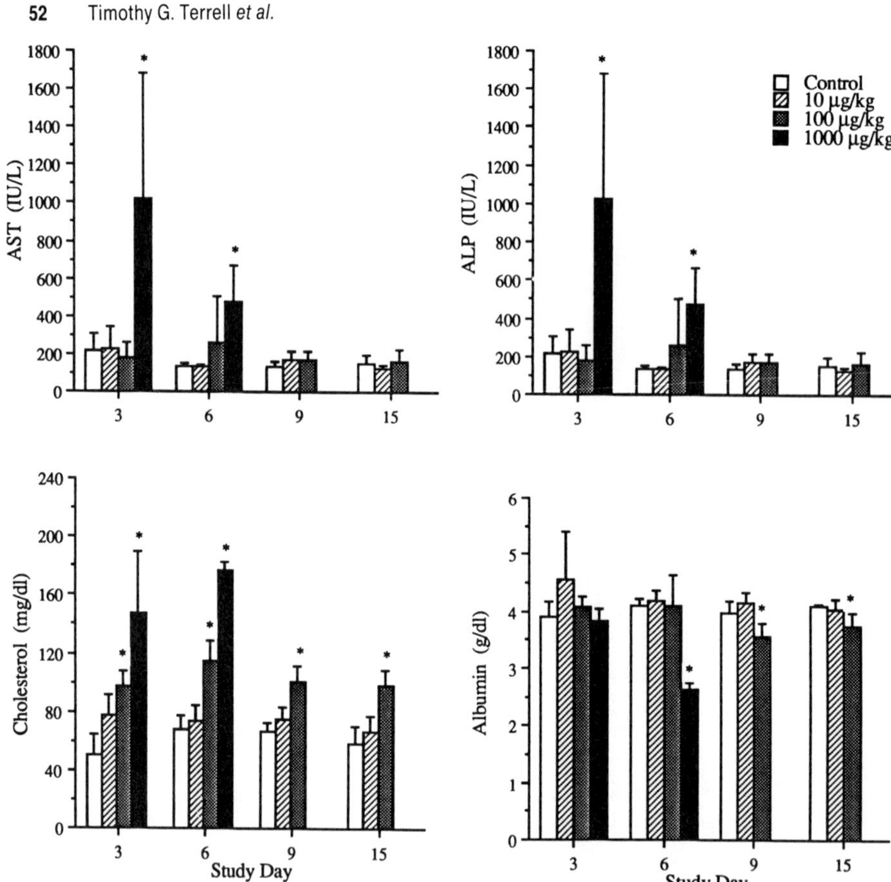

Fig. 4. Mean serum chemistry values for rats treated intravenously with rHuTGF-β1 for 14 days. Data for male animals only are shown, but similar results were present in females. High-dose animals were sacrificed after 5 days of treatment. Statistically significant differences when compared to controls of same sex using the Student's *t* test are indicated (*, $p < 0.05$).

severity. The marked decrease in size of the liver was due to a widespread centrilobular degeneration and removal of hepatocytes. This lesion correlated with serum increases in liver enzymes and bilirubin levels consistent with hepatocellular necrosis and cholestasis. Individual hepatic lobules were markedly decreased in size (Fig. 6). The normal hepatic architecture was disrupted and, due to the loss of hepatocytes in the centrilobular area, there was an increased density of reticulum fibers in these area. Biliary hyperplasia and periportal fibrosis was present in high-dose animals. Individual hepatocytes were enlarged with karyomegaly and increased cytoplasm (Fig. 7), and the number of mitotic figures in the hepatocytes was markedly increased at

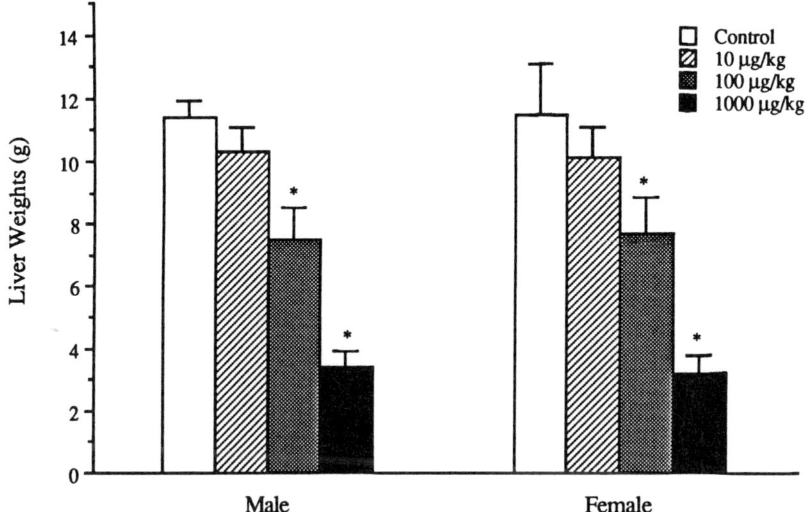

Fig. 5. Mean liver weights for rats treated intravenously with rHuTGF-β1 for 14 days. Statistically significant differences when compared to controls of same sex using the Student's *t* test are indicated (*, $p < 0.05$).

all dose levels. An increase in mononuclear inflammatory cells was observed in periportal areas.

Thymic atrophy characterized by decreased thickness of the cortex due to depletion of cortical thymocytes (Fig. 8) was observed at the high-dose level. Mild lymphoid depletion was also observed in spleen and lymph nodes.

Treatment-related changes in the kidney included a slight hypercellularity of the glomeruli and increased vacuolization and numbers of mitotic figures in proximal tubular epithelial cells (Fig. 9). These renal changes were observed primarily in the high-dose group. A minimal to mild proliferative nonsuppurative inflammatory lesion was present in the heart valves of most mid- and high-dose animals (Fig. 10).

Very marked endosteal new bone formation was observed in all high-dose animals after 5 days of treatment (Fig. 11). This lesion was associated with hyperplasia of osteoblasts and increased formation of extracellular matrix (Fig. 12). Similar but milder bone changes were observed in some animals at the mid-dose level.

All high-dose animals had moderate degranulation and degeneration of β cells at the periphery of the islets of Langerhan in the pancreas (Fig. 13). Acinar cells in the pancreas of several high-dose animals demonstrated a depletion of basilar basophilic cytoplasmic staining. The significance of this latter observation is not known. Diffuse, mild gastritis and typhlitis with moderate submucosal edema were also observed in many of the high-dose

Table III. Incidence and Severity of Selected Histopathological Lesions in Rats Treated with rHuTGF-β1 Intravenously for 14 Days

Tissue/lesion	Control	10	100	1000
			Dose (μg/kg/day)	
Thymus				
Lymphoid depletion	$-$[a]	+ (2/10)	+ (3/10)[b]	++++ (8/8)
Lymphoid necrosis	$-$	$-$	$-$	++ (8/8)
Liver				
Hepatocellular degeneration	$-$	P[c] (6/10)	P (8/10)	P (10/10)
Increased mitotic index	$-$	+++ (10/10)	+++ (10/10)	+++ (10/10)
Oval cell proliferation	$-$	$-$	++ (10/10)	++++ (10/10)
Fibrosis	$-$	$-$	+ (5/10)	+++ (10/10)
Biliary hyperplasia	$-$	$-$	$-$	+++ (10/10)
Kidney				
Epithelial hyperplasia	$-$	$-$	P (1/10)	P (9/10)
Glomerulosclerosis	$\pm$ (4/10)	$\pm$ (2/10)	+ (3/10)	++ (8/10)
Bone				
Enostosis		$-$	+ (6/10)	+++ (8/8)
Osteoblast hyperplasia	+ (1/10)	+ (4/10)	++ (9/10)	++++ (8/8)
Heart				
Valvulitis	$-$	+ (1/3)	+ (1/3)	+++ (8/10)
Pancreas				
Islet cell degeneration	$-$	$-$	P (2/10)	P (8/8)
Gastrointestinal tract				
Gastritis	$\pm$ (2/10)	$-$	$\pm$ (2/10)	++ (5/8)
Typhlitis	$-$	+ (1/10)	+ (1/10)	++ (7/8)
Injection vein (tail)				
Perivascular inflammation	+ (10/10)	++ (10/10)	++ (10/10)	+++ (8/8)
Fibrosis	$-$	+++ (10/10)	+++ (10/10)	++ (8/8)
Anesthetic injection site				
Hyperproliferative fibroplasia	$-$	+++ (2/10)	+++ (3/10)	++++ (6/8)

[a] Lesion severity grades: $-$, not present; +, minimal; ++, mild; +++, moderate; ++++, severe.

[b] Number of animals with lesion present/number of animals examined.

[c] P, Present.

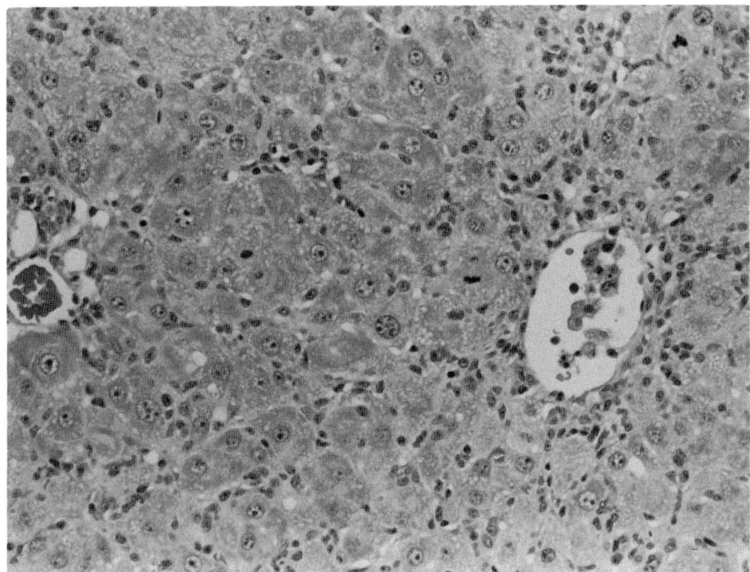

Fig. 6. Liver from rat treated intravenously with 1000 µg/kg/day of rHuTGF-β1 for 5 days. There is marked reduction in size of the hepatic lobule, with disruption of hepatic cords. Hematoxylin and eosin (×160).

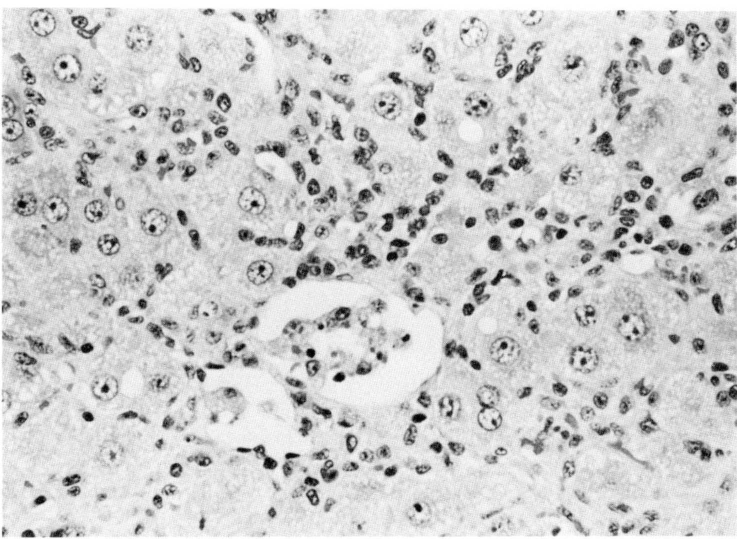

Fig. 7. Higher magnification of the same liver showing hepatocellular hypertrophy with karyomegaly and mononuclear inflammatory cell infiltration. Central vein contains dislodged hepatocytes in its lumen. Hematoxylin and eosin (×380).

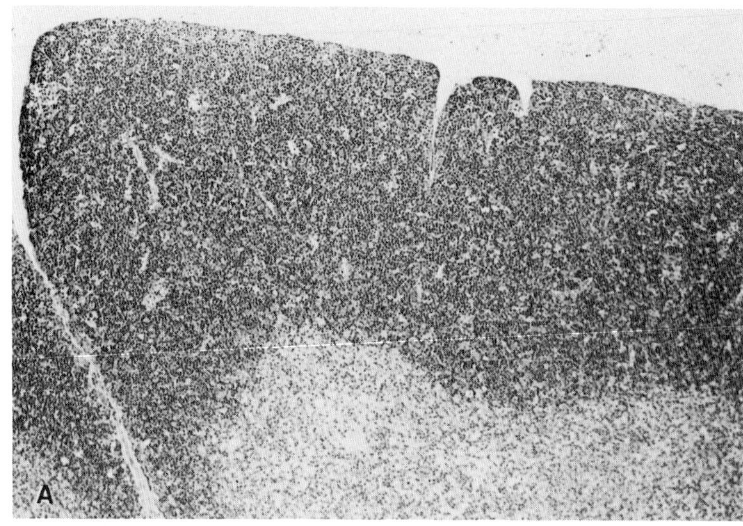

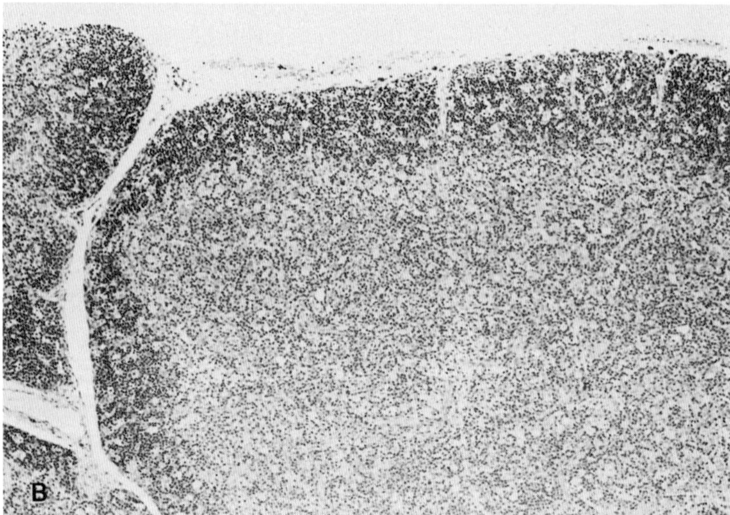

Fig. 8. Photomicrograph of thymus from rats. (a) Control rat showing the normal cellularity and structure of thymic lobule. (b) Rat treated intravenously with 1000 μg/kg/day of rHuTGF-β1 for 5 days; there is marked thymic atrophy with depletion of cortical thymocytes. Hematoxylin and eosin ($\times$100).

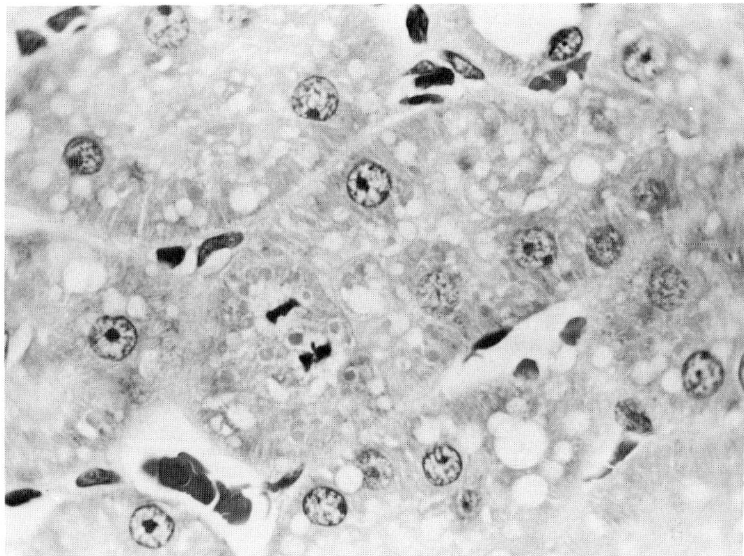

Fig. 9. Kidney from rat treated intravenously with 1000 μg/kg/day of rHuTGF-β1 for 5 days showing vacuolation of proximal tubular epithelial cells, with a mitotic figure present in one cell. Hematoxylin and eosin (×1000).

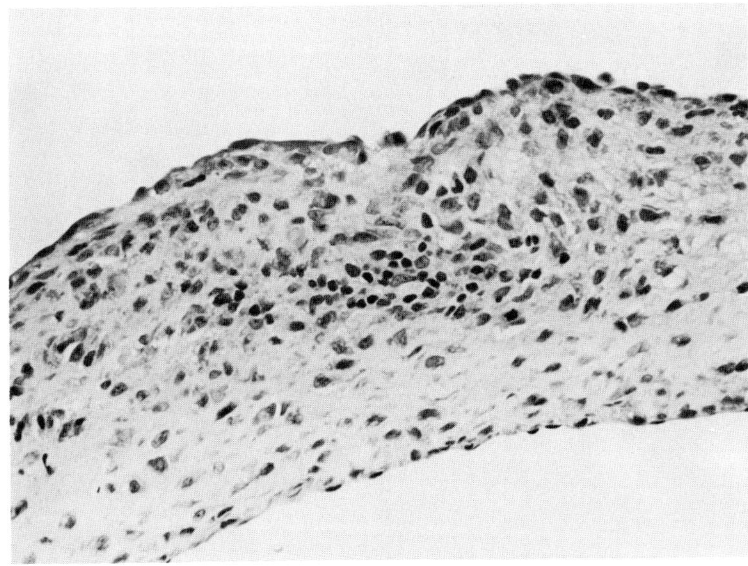

Fig. 10. Heart valve from rat treated intravenously with 1000 μg/kg/day of rHuTGF-β1 for 5 days showing focal area of nonsuppurative inflammation. Hematoxylin and eosin (×380).

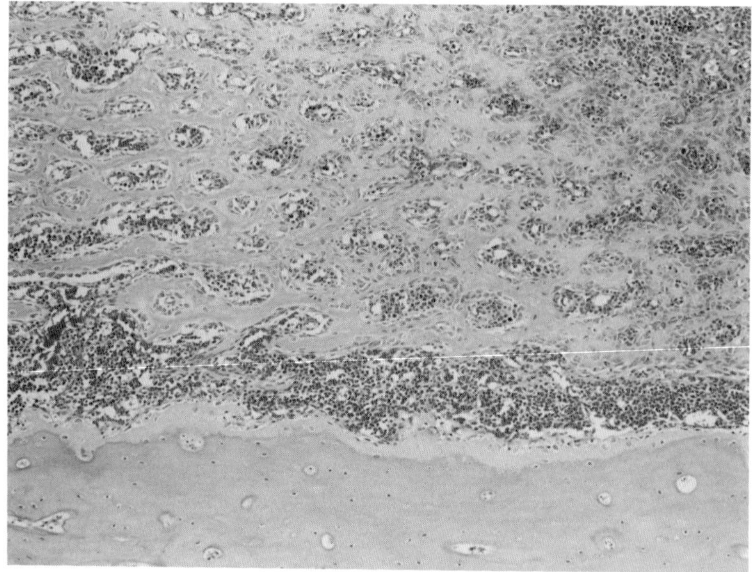

Fig. 11. Enosteal bone proliferation in femur of rat treated intravenously with 1000 μg/kg/day of rHuTGF-β1 for 5 days. Hematoxylin and eosin ($\times$100).

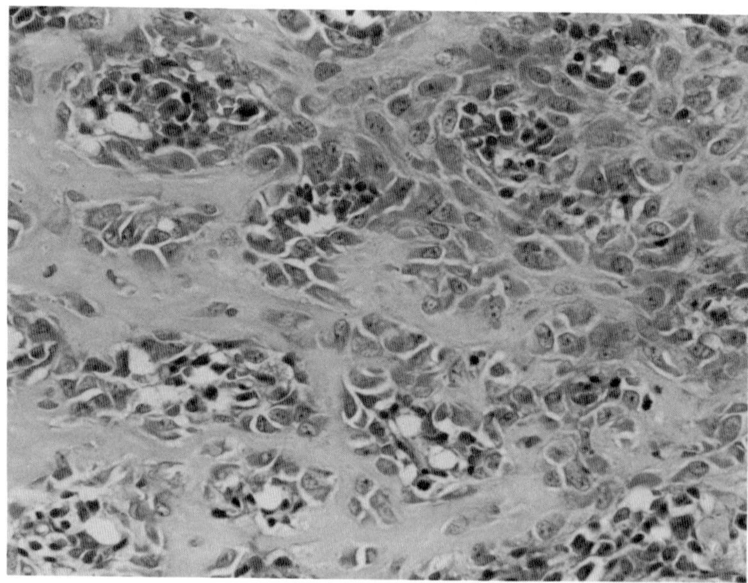

Fig. 12. Higher magnification of Fig. 11 showing osteoblast hyperplasia and increased formation of extracellular matrix. Hematoxylin and eosin ($\times$380).

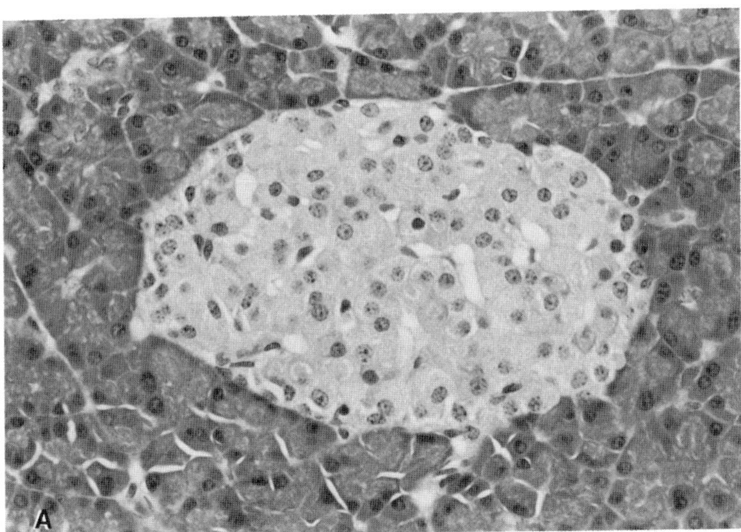

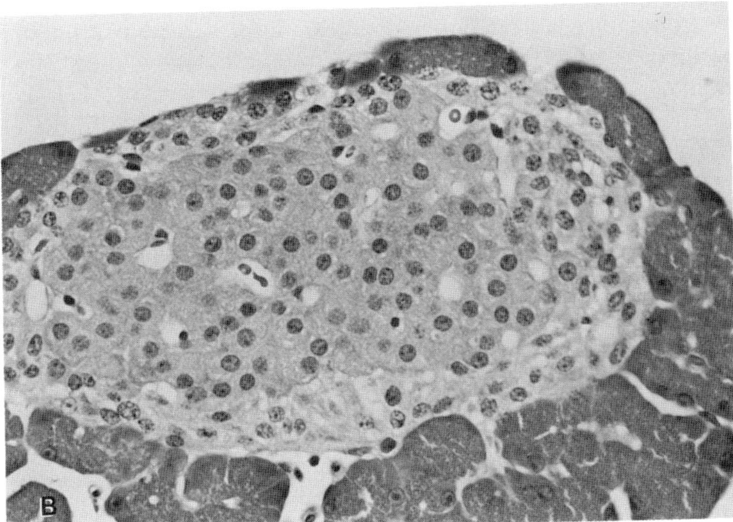

Fig. 13. Photomicrograph of pancreas from rats. (a) Control rat showing normal islet structure. Hematoxylin and eosin (×380). (b) Pancreas from rat treated intravenously with 1000 μg/kg/day of rHuTGF-β1 intravenously for 5 days. There is a zone of degeneration and vacuolation of β cells at the periphery of the islet and diffuse atrophy of acinar cells. Hematoxylin and eosin (×380).

group animals (Fig. 14). Animals were anesthetized with intramuscular injections of ketamine hydrochloride for blood collection at intervals throughout the study. Ketamine is irritating and produces tissue necrosis, inflammation, and fibrosis following intramuscular injection (Smiler *et al.*, 1990). In animals treated intravenously with rHuTGF-β1, there was an unusual hyperproliferative fibroblastic (Fig. 15) response associated with the healing anesthetic site lesion.

Perivascular changes at the injection site (lateral tail vein) of rHuTGF-β1-treated animals were characterized by increased inflammation, fibrosis, and bone proliferation in the adjacent coccygeal vertebrae.

In order to evaluate more fully the potential effects of systemic exposure to rHuTGF-β1 at lower doses than those utilized in the pilot study, a 4-week subchronic intravenous toxicity study in rats was conducted with doses of 0.125, 1.25, or 12.5 μg/kg/day of the rHuTGF-β1 produced in the CHO cell line. The selection of doses for this study was based on several considerations. The planned clinical use for promotion of wound healing involved topical application of the rHuTGF-β1 to open wounds. Preclinical pharmacology studies have shown that radioiodinated rHuTGF-β1 is poorly absorbed from topical application to open wounds (T. Zioncheck, unpublished observations), so low systemic exposure would be anticipated. This study was designed to examine the potential target organ effects of rHuTGF-β1 at a level of systemic exposure that would be more supportive of the clinical situation. Additionally, the formulations produced from the A293 cells and the CHO cells were not equivalent, and it is difficult to predict what doses were actually achieved in the pilot study. Animals were treated by single daily intravenous bolus injections for 28 days, and a subset of animals in the control and high-dose groups was allowed a 4-week recovery period. All doses were well tolerated and there were no deaths or significant clinical signs of toxicity. There as a slight reduction in erythroid parameters (erythrocytes, hematocrit, and hemoglobin) in animals at the high dose (Fig. 16). Liver weights were slightly decreased at the high dose (Fig. 17). This change was accompanied by mildly increased serum levels of the liver enzymes AST, ALT, and ALP, and decreased albumin (Fig. 18). There were no treatment-related histopathological changes in the liver or any other organs, and the changes observed in clinical pathology parameters were reversed after a 4-week recovery period. No antibody response to rHuTGF-β1 was detected.

III. DISCUSSION

Recombinant human TGF-β1 presented several unique considerations for safety assessment to support clinical testing. Unlike many of the cytokines and growth factors, it is not limited in the range of species in which it has

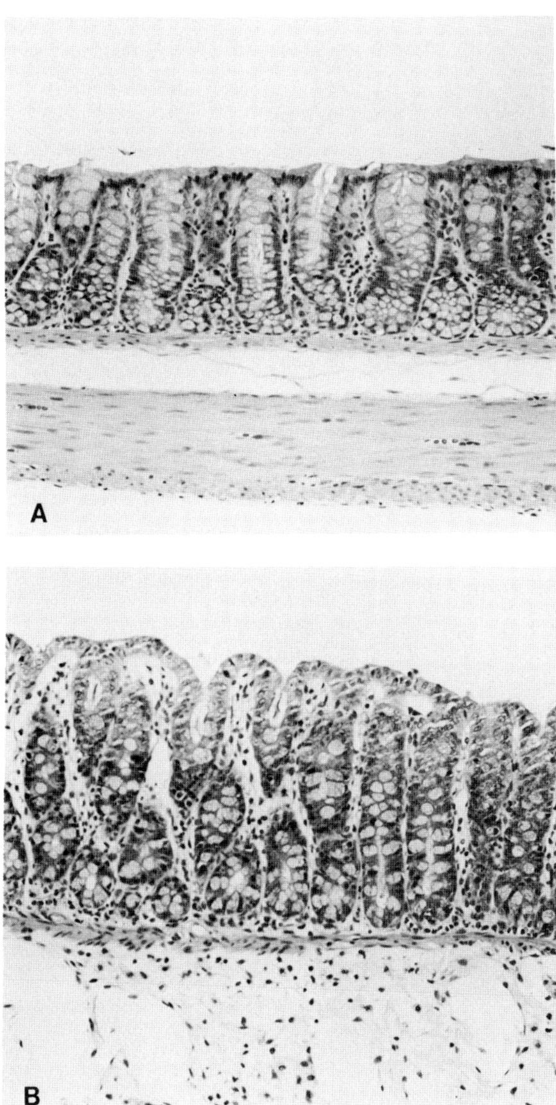

Fig. 14. Photomicrograph of cecum from rats. (a) Control rat showing normal structure. Hematoxylin and eosin (×160). (b) Cecum from rat treated intravenously with 1000 μg/kg/day of rHuTGF-β1 for 5 days showing diffuse typhlitis and submucosal edema. Hematoxylin and eosin (×160).

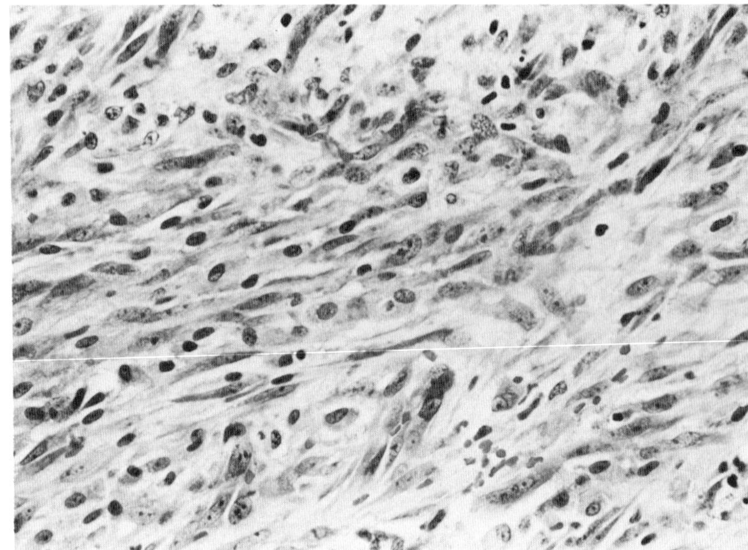

Fig. 15. Site of ketamine hydrochloride injection in a rat treated intravenously with 1000 μg/kg/day of rHuTGF-β1 for 5 days showing hyperproliferative fibroblastic response. Hematoxylin and eosin ($\times$380).

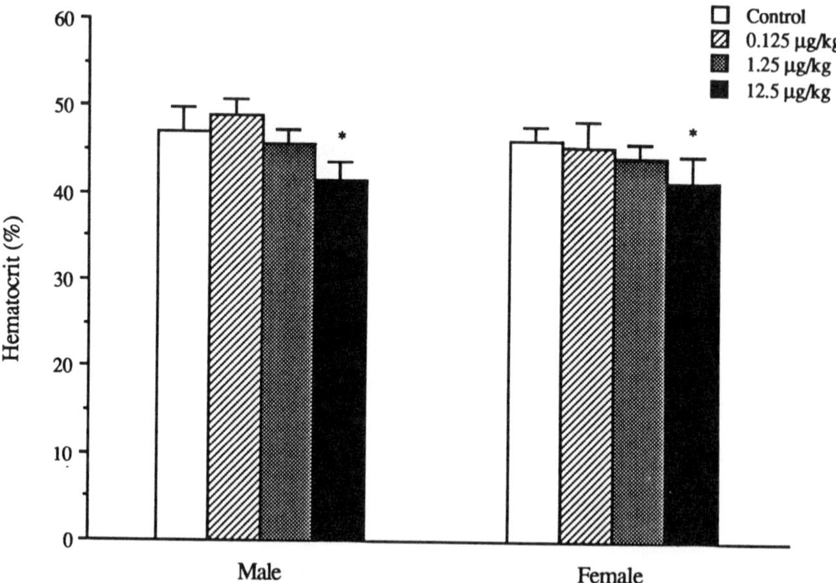

Fig. 16. Mean hematocrits for rats treated intravenously with rHuTGF-β1 for 4 weeks. Statistically significant differences when compared to controls of same sex using the Student's t test are indicated ($*$, $p < 0.05$).

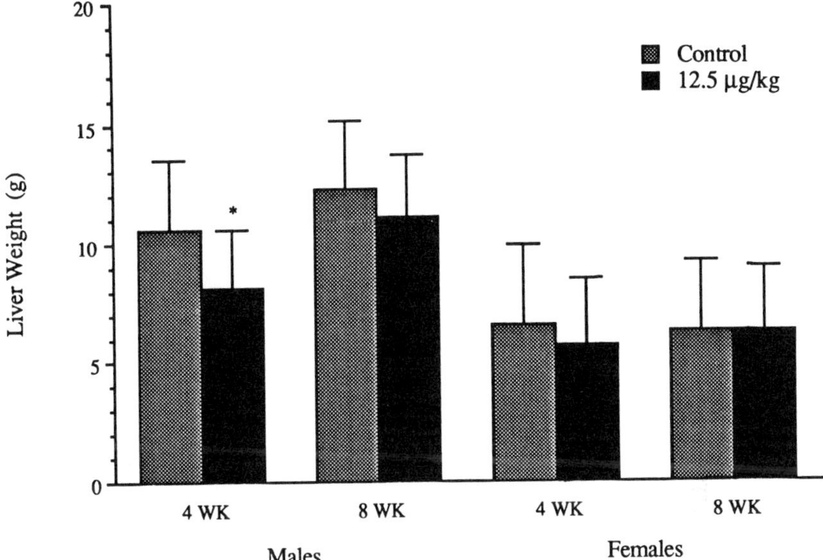

Fig. 17. Mean liver weights for rats treated intravenously with rHuTGF-β1 for 4 weeks and after a 4-week posttreatment recovery period. Statistically significant differences when compared to controls of same sex using the Student's *t* test are indicated (∗, $p < 0.05$).

biological activity. In fact, TGF-β is extremely well conserved across species and there is greater than 99% identity in the amino acid sequence of TGF-β between several mammalian species tested. The rHuTGF-β1 has activity in several animal model systems, including the rabbit and rat. Also, because of the high degree of homology between species, antibody responses to exogenous sources of the polypeptide are unlikely to present a significant problem in safety studies. However, because of the many biological activities of TGF-β1 and the widespread tissue distribution of the TGF-β receptor, it may be expected to have diverse and numerous target organ effects. This is, in fact, what was observed with systemic exposure to high doses of rHuTGF-β1. Rats treated intravenously with 100–1000 μg/kg/day developed lesions in liver, bone, kidney, heart, thymus, pancreas, stomach, cecum, at the injection vein, and in skeletal muscle at the site of anesthetic injection. The pathogenic mechanism for the majority of lesions in these organs can be predicted on the basis of known activities of TGF-β from *in vitro* and *in vivo* studies. The relative severity and rapidity with which some of the changes (such as the hepatic involution and enostosis) developed was remarkable. TGF-β is a potent mitogenic factor for osteoblasts and stimulates the formation of new bone in *ex vivo* systems (Centrella *et al.,* 1987; Robey *et al.,* 1987). Osteoblast hyperplasia and deposition of extracellular matrix were the principal

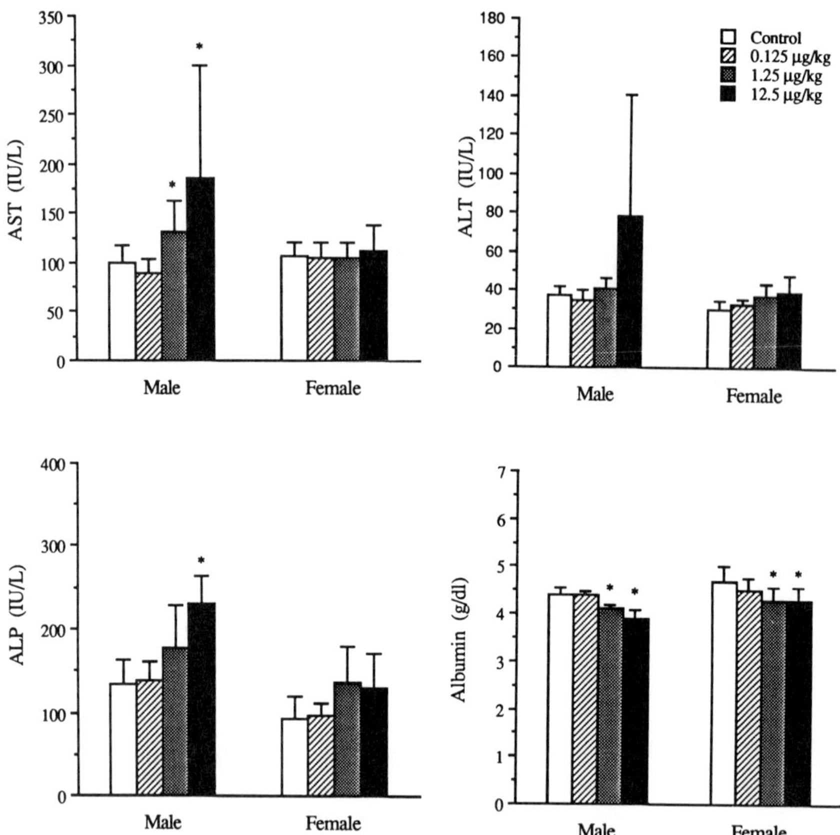

Fig. 18. Mean serum chemistry values for rats treated intravenously with rHuTGF-β1 for 4 weeks. Statistically significant differences when compared to controls of same sex using the Student's *t* test are indicated (∗, $p < 0.05$).

responses that led to the enostosis in the long bones. It was not possible to determine if the matrix was mineralized because the specimens were subjected to decalcification procedures during processing. The severity and extent of the bone reaction would suggest that osteoblasts are very responsive to systemic administration of the molecule. This response may be beneficial in some circumstances, such as fracture repair, but may represent a dose-limiting adverse reaction in other circumstances.

The hepatic involution was also a dramatic response to the high-dose systemic administration of rHuTGF-β1. Rats receiving 1000 μg/kg/day had a 70% reduction in liver mass after only 5 days of treatment. Histologically, there was very little evidence of hepatocellular degeneration or necrosis; however, the decrease in liver mass was due to a loss of hepatocytes from lobules, and therefore reflected the result of hepatocellular necrosis. These observations were supported by the serum chemistry changes. The mechanism of the rHuTGF-β1-induced hepatocellular necrosis and degeneration is not evident. TGF-β is a potent inhibitor of hepatocyte DNA synthesis (Nakamura *et al.*, 1985; McMahon *et al.*, 1987) and may function as a physiological regulator of liver regeneration (Braun *et al.*, 1988; Mead and Fausto, 1989). It is possible that, at high enough levels, the cytostatic effect of TGF-β on hepatocytes may be cytotoxic. An apparent paradoxical observation, because TGF-β is an inhibitor of hepatocyte proliferation, was the presence of high numbers of mitotic figures in hepatocytes in the livers and kidneys of the rHuTGF-β1-treated animals. This probably was not a direct effect of the rHuTGF-β1, but a secondary change, possibly in response to other mediators, such as hepatocyte growth factor (Lindroos *et al.*, 1991).

Thymic atrophy, as observed at the high-dose levels, is consistent with the immunosuppressive effects of TGF-β (Wallick *et al.*, 1990) and its inhibition of lymphocyte proliferation (Russell *et al.*, 1988). The mild depression of hematocrit and erythroid parameters in peripheral blood may be due to the inhibitory effects of TGF-β1 on hematopoietic cells (Keller *et al.*, 1989). Other lesions observed in rHuTGF-β1-treated rats included gastrointestinal tract inflammation and edema and degeneration of β cells in pancreatic islets. The mechanism of induction of these changes is not apparent based on known activities of the molecule.

An unusual hyperproliferative fibroblastic response was observed at the site of ketamine injection in animals treated intravenously with rHuTGF-β1. As mentioned previously, ketamine is irritating and produces tissue necrosis, inflammation, and fibrosis following intramuscular injection (Smiler *et al.*, 1990). The systemic administration of rHuTGF-β1 resulted in an exaggeration of the fibroplasia associated with this normal healing response at the local site. This reaction is consistent with the mitogenic activity of TGF-β in fibroblasts, and it appeared that fibroblasts proliferating in response to a local injury were more sensitive to the mitogenic activity of the rHuTGF-β1 than were fibroblasts at other noninjury sites in the body.

Because the proposed therapeutic application for the rHuTGF-β1 is for topical application to promote wound healing, safety studies were conducted in which the test material was applied to wound sites to mimic the clinical exposure. High-dose dermal application resulted in local effects at the wound sites without systemic toxicity. The lack of systemic effects can be attributed to the low level of absorption of rHuTGF-β1 from the wound sites. There was no formation of antibody to rHuTGF-β1 in rats or rabbits treated topically. The lack of an antibody response may be due to either the high degree of conservation of this peptide across species, or to the low level of systemic exposure following topical treatment. In rabbits, the topical application of rHuTGF-β1 resulted in impairment of the wound healing. This contrasts with earlier studies in which rHuTGF-β1 was shown to enhance wound closure and healing (Beck *et al.,* 1990). The apparent conflicting results is probably the result of dosage. The doses used in the toxicity study were approximately 80 times higher than the dose used in the efficacy studies. Promotion of wound healing would be consistent with known activities of TGF-β, which results in stimulation of formation of granulation tissue (Roberts *et al.,* 1986). The delayed healing observed in the toxicity study was attributed to a failure of the epithelium to proliferate over the open wound, resulting in wound closure. Topically applied rHuTGF-β1 is retained at the site in the dimeric form for up to 48 hr after application (T. Zioncheck, unpublished observations), and at high doses may result in direct inhibition of epithelial cell proliferation (Moses *et al.,* 1990). The fact that similar lesions were not observed in the multidose study in rabbits, wherein the high dose was lower than that used in the single-dose study, also supports the conclusion that the differential response was a function of dose.

IV. SUMMARY

The systemic administration of high doses of rHuTGF-β1 to rats produced a spectrum of lesions in multiple target tissues, including liver, bone, kidney, heart, thymus, pancreas, stomach, cecum, at the injection vein, and in skeletal muscle at the site of anesthetic injection. The majority of these lesions can be attributed to known biological activities of TGF-β1. High-dose dermal application resulted in local effects at the wound sites without systemic toxicity.

Acknowledgments

The material reviewed includes data from studies conducted to support registration of rHuTGF-β1. The authors wish to thank D. Liggitt, S. Beck, A. Ammann, and E. Amento at Genentech, and M. Palazollo, K. MacKenzie, R. Hall, R. Busch, R. Alsaker, and J. Carter at Hazleton Wisconsin for their individual contributions to these studies.

References

Ammann, A. J., Beck, L. S., DeGuzman, L., Hirabayashi, S. E., Lee, W. P., McFatridge, L., Mustoe, T. A., Nguyen, T., and Xu, Y. (1990). *Ann. N.Y. Acad. Sci.* **593,** 124–134.

Assoian, K., Komoriya, A., Meyers, C. A., Miller, D. M., and Sporn, M. B. (1983). *J. Biol. Chem.* **258,** 7155–7160.

Beck, L. S., Chen, T. L., Mikalauski, P., and Ammann, A. J. (1990). *Growth Factors* **3,** 267–275.

Braun, L., Mead, J. E., Panzica, M., Mikumo, R., Bell, G. I., and Fausto, N. (1988). *Proc. Natl. Acad. Sci. U.S.A.* **85,** 1539–1543.

Centrella, M., McCarthy, T. L., and Canalis, E. (1987). *J. Biol. Chem.* **262,** 2869–2874.

De Larco, J. E., and Todaro, G. J. (1978). *Proc. Natl. Acad. Sci. U.S. A.* **75,** 4001–4005.

Derynck, R., Jarrett, J. A., Chen, E. Y., Eaton, D. H., Bell, J. R., Assoian, R. K., Roberts, A. B., Sporn, M. B., and Goeddel, D. V. (1985). *Nature (London)* **316,** 701–705.

Derynck, R., Jarrett, J. A., Chen, E. Y., and Goeddel, D. V. (1986). *J. Biol. Chem.* **261,** 4377–4379.

Derynck, R., Rhee, L., Chen, E. Y., and Van Tilburg, A. (1987). *Nucleic Acid Res.* **15,** 3188–3189.

Heine, U. I., Munoz, E. F., Flanders, K. C., Ellingworth, L. R., Lam, H. Y. P., Thompson, N. L., Roberts, A. B., and Sporn, M. B. (1987). *J. Cell Biol.* **105,** 2861–2876.

Keller, J. R., Sing, G. K., Ellingsworth, L. R., and Ruscetti, F. W. (1989). *J. Cell. Biochem.* **39,** 175–184.

LaMarre, J., Wollenberg, G. K., Gonias, S. L., and Hayes, M. A. (1991). *Lab. Invest.* **65,** 3–14.

Lehnert, S. A., and Akhurst, R. J. (1988). *Development* **104,** 263–273.

Lindroos, P. M., Zarnegar, R., and Michalopoulos, G. K. (1991). *Hepatology* **13,** 743–749.

Massagué, J. (1987). *Cell* **49,** 437–438.

Massagué, J. (1990). *In* "The Transforming Growth Factor-β Family" (G. E. PAlade, B. M. Alberts, and J. A. Spudich, eds.), Vol. 6, pp. 597–641. Annu. Rev., Palo Alto, California.

Massagué, J., Kelly, B., and Mottola, C. (1985). *J. Biol. Chem.* **260,** 4551–4554.

McMahon, J. B., Richards, W. L., del Campo, A. A., Song, M. K. H., and Thorgeirsson, S. S. (1987). *Cancer Res.* **46,** 4665–4671.

Mead, J. E., and Fausto, N. (1989). *Proc. Natl. Acad. Sci. U.S.A.* **86,** 1558–1562.

Moses, H. L. (1990). *In* "Growth Factors: From Genes to Clinical Applications" (S. R. Vicki, ed.), pp. 141–155. Raven, New York.

Moses, H. L., Branum, E. B., Proper, J. A., and Robinson, R. A. (1981). *Cancer Res.* **41,** 2842–2848.

Moses, H. L., Yang, E. Y., and Pietenpol, J. A. (1990). *Cell* **63,** 245–247.

Mustoe, T. A., Pierce, G. F., Thomason, A., Gramates, P., Sporn, M. B., and Deuel, T. F. (1987). *Science* **237,** 1333–1336.

Nakamura, T., Tomita, Y., Hirai, R., Yamaoka, K., Kaji, K., and Ichihara, A. (1985). *Biochem. Biophys. Res. Commun.* **133,** 1042–1050.

Roberts, A. B., and Sporn, M. B. (1990). *In* "Handbook of Experimental Pharmacology: Peptide Growth Factors and Their Receptors" (M. B. Sporn and A. B. Roberts, eds.), Vol. 95, pp. 419–472. Springer-Verlag, Berlin.

Roberts, A. B., Anzano, M. A., Lamb, L. C., Smith, J. M., and Sporn, M. B. (1981). *Proc. Natl. Acad. Sci. U.S.A.* **78,** 5339–5343.

Roberts, A. B., Sporn, M. B., Assoian, R. K., Smith, J. M., Roche, N. S., Wakefield, L. M., Heine, U. I., Liotta, L. A., Falanga, V., Kehrl, J. H., and Fauci, A. S. (1986). *Proc. Natl. Acad. Sci. U.S.A.* **83,** 4167–4171.

Robey, P. G., Young, M. F., Flanders, K. C., Roche, N. S., Kondaiah, P., Reddi, A. H., Termine, J. D., Sporn, M. B., and Roberts, A. B. (1987). *J. Cell Biol.* **105,** 457–463.

Russell, W. E., Coffey, R. J., Jr., Ouellette, A. J., and Moses, H. L. (1988). *Proc. Natl. Acad. Sci. U.S.A.* **85,** 5126–5130.

Silberstein, G. B., and Daniel, C. W. (1987). *Science* **237,** 291–293.

Smiler, K. L., Stein, S., Hrapkiewicz, K. L., and Hiben, J. R. (1990). *Lab. Anim. Sci.* **40,** 60–64.

Sporn, M. B., and Roberts, A. B. (1987). *J. Cell Biol.* **105,** 1039–1045.

Sporn, M. B., Roberts, A. B., Wakefield, L. M., and de Crombrugghe, B. (1987). *J. Cell Biol.* **105,** 1039–1045.

Wahl, S. M., Hunt, D. A., Wakefield, L. M., McCartney-Francis, N., Wahl, L. M., Roberts, A. B., and Sporn, M. B. (1987). *Proc. Natl. Acad. Sci. U.S.A.* **84,** 5788–5792.

Wakefield, L. M., Smith, D. M., Masui, T., Harris, C. C., and Sporn, M. B. (1987). *J. Cell Biol.* **105,** 965–975.

Wallick, S. C., Figari, I. A., Morris, R. E., Levinson, A. D., and Palladino, M. A. (1990). *J. Exp. Med.* **172,** 1777–1784.

Wilcox, J. N., and Derynck, R. (1988). *Mol. Cell. Biol.* **8,** 3415–3422.

Pathology Induced by Leukemia Inhibitory Factor

Bernhard Ryffel

Institut für Toxikologie
Eidgenössischen Technischen Hochschule
Universität Zürich
CH-8603 Schwerzenbach/Zürich, Switzerland

I. INTRODUCTION

Leukemia inhibitory factor (LIF) was originally identified as a factor inducing macrophage differentiation of the murine myeloid leukemia cell line M1 (Metcalf *et al.,* 1988). LIF induces proliferation of hematopoietic stem cells and the DA cell line (Fletcher *et al.,* 1990; Moreau *et al.,* 1988). Evidence of broad actions of LIF have recently been shown, including bone regeneration (Reid *et al.,* 1990), induction of acute-phase responses in hepatocytes (Baumann and Wong, 1989), nerve differentiation (Yamamori *et al.,* 1989), inhibition of adipogenesis (Mori *et al.,* 1989), and suppression of embryonic stem cell differentiation (Gough *et al.,* 1989; for review of biological activity, see Gough and Williams, 1989).

LIF is produced by a number of different tumor cell lines, antigen- and mitogen-stimulated lymphoid cells. Molecular clones encoding murine and human LIF have been isolated and the proteins expressed (Gearing *et al.,* 1987; Gough *et al.,* 1988; Moreau *et al.,* 1988). The cDNA encodes a protein of 20 kDa containing 179 amino acids; the mature protein has a molecular mass between 38 and 67 kDa due to extensive and variable glycosylation. The role of the carbohydrate moiety is unclear because nonglycosylated *Escherichia coli*-derived LIF is highly active. The homology of murine and human LIF is 79% at the protein level (Gough *et al.,* 1988).

The biological activity of LIF has some resemblance to that of IL-6. IL-6 causes hematopoietic stem cell and megakaryocyte progenitor cell proliferation, neuronal differentiation, and bone regeneration; it induces the hepatic synthesis of acute-phase proteins and is a potent inflammatory mediator (Hirano *et al.,* 1990). Toward understanding the diverse action of LIF at the molecular level, the recent discovery of the structure of the LIF receptor and its homology to the IL-6 and granulocyte colong-stimulating factor (G-CSF) receptor may be important (Gearing *et al.,* 1991; Hibi *et al.,* 1990).

A brief examination of the biological activity of LIF is presented here to explain the *in vivo* effects of the recombinant protein as tested in mice and nonhuman primates.

II. PATHOLOGY INDUCED BY LIF

A. Mice

The *in vivo* effects of LIF were investigated in mice engrafted with FDC-P1 cells producing high levels of LIF (Metcalf and Gearing, 1989a,b). DBA2J mice subjected to whole-body irradiation were injected with 10^6 LIF-producing FDC-P1 cells. LIF-producing cells were observed in the bone marrow, spleen, and lymph nodes; high serum levels of LIF were detected in the mice. These mice developed a fatal syndrome with cachexia, excess bone formation, and multiple calcifications. Subcutaneous and abdominal fat loss, atrophy of liver and kidney, and distinct body weight loss were found in LIF-transfected animals. In the bone, an increased osteoblastic activity resulted in excess new bone formation and obliteration of the marrow space, resulting in myelosclerosis. Calcification, possibly a metastatic type, was found in the myocardium and skeletal muscle. The lymphoid follicles in spleen and lymph nodes as well as in the thymus were atrophic. The pancreas showed signs of necrosis and inflammation. The results of these investigations suggest that LIF is toxic, causes cachexia, and has marked effects on osteoblast activity and calcium metabolism (Metcalf and Gearing, 1989a,b).

Metcalf and co-workers also reported on the effects of recombinant murine LIF injected into mice (Metcalf *et al.,* 1990). *Escherichia coli*-derived LIF was given in daily doses of up to 6 μg/mouse over 2 weeks to DBA/2 and C3H/HeJ mice. At this high-dose level ($\sim$300 μg/kg), LIF caused signs of general toxicity with body weight loss, loss of body fat, behavioral changes, and thymic atrophy. Bone marrow cellularity was decreased and signs of an acute-phase response were evident (increased erythrocyte sedimentation rates and decreased albumin levels). Megakaryocyte and progenitor cell numbers were increased both in the bone marrow and in the spleen and were associated with dose-related increases in platelet numbers.

Preliminary results in rats treated with murine LIF up to doses of 100 μg/kg did not reveal major adverse effects (B. Ryffel, unpublished observations).

In mice, LIF at high doses caused cachexia, an acute-phase response, and also had effects on bone and hematopoiesis *in vivo.* Whether the beneficial effect of LIF on megakaryocyte maturation might be used clinically in the treatment of thrombocytopenia depends on whether these effects are separable from the generalized effects of this growth factor.

B. Nonhuman Primates

The biological effects of LIF were investigated in rhesus monkeys, which received daily subcutaneous doses up to 50 μg/kg over 14 days (P. Mayer, in preparation). Within 3 days, recombinant LIF caused an acute-phase response, even at the low dose of 5 μg/kg. At the high dose, body weight loss was found. Furthermore, LIF induced a slight increase in total leukocyte counts, essentially an increase of neutrophils, and a twofold increase in normal platelet counts. Elevation of platelet counts occurred after 10 days and was reversible on cessation of treatment. Bone marrow cellularity and megakaryocyte number were not changed by LIF administration. No further information on general and organ toxicity is available from this study.

III. DISCUSSION

In common with other cytokines, especially IL-6 and TNF, LIF has a broad spectrum of biological activities. LIF caused an immediate acute-phase response that is associated with cachexia. Effects on hematopoietic progenitors as described in pharmacological studies were not investigated in detail in these *in vivo* studies; however, the main effect observed in mice and primates is a stimulation of megakaryopoiesis, resulting in increased blood platelet counts. The specificity of LIF is not limited to this, however, as LIF activity on bone regeneration, adipose tissue, and nerve differentiation has been shown.

Specific binding of LIF has been demonstrated in diverse tissues (Hilton *et al.,* 1988). Toward a molecular understanding of the diverse actions the of LIF, recent cloning of the LIF receptor may prove helpful (Gearing *et al.,* 1991). The human LIF receptor is related to the gp130 component of the IL-6 receptor and to the G-CSF receptor; the transmembrane and cytoplasmic regions of the LIF receptor and the signal-transducing component of IL-6R, gp130, are closely related (Taga *et al.,* 1989). This relationship suggests common signal transduction pathways for the two receptor systems and might explain the similar biological profiles of the two ligands.

IV. SUMMARY

Leukemia inhibitory factor is a glycoprotein growth and differentiation factor with pleiotropic activity. LIF has potent effects on the hematopoietic system, including megakaryocyte progenitor cells. In addition, LIF has bone regeneration activity, induces cachexia and acute-phase response in hepatocytes, and inhibits adipogenesis, to mention the more important activities. *In vivo* LIF treatment in monkeys and rodents was followed by signs of general toxicity, cachexia, acute-phase reaction, and stimulation of hematopoiesis. The safety margin for possible therapeutic effects on hematopoiesis seems to be very narrow.

References

Baumann, H., and Wong, G. G. (1989). *J. Immunol.* **143**, 1163.

Fletcher, F. A., Williams, D. E., Maliszewski, C., Anderson, D., Rives, M., and Belmont, J. W. (1990). *Blood* **76**, 1098.

Gearing, D. P., Gough, N. M., King, J. A., Hilton, D. J., Nicola, N. A., Simpson, R. J., Nice, E. C., Kelso, A., and Metcalf, D. (1987). *EMBO J.* **6**, 3995.

Gearing, D. P., Thut, C. J., VandenBos, T., Gimpel, St. D., Delaney, P. B., King, J., Price, V., Cosman, D., and Beckmann, M. P. (1991). *EMBO J.* **10**, 2839.

Gough, N. M., and Williams, R. L. (1989). *Cancer Cells* **1**, 77.

Gough, N. M., Gearing, D. P., King, J. A., Willson, T. A., Hilton, D. J., Nicola, N. A., and Metcalf, D. (1988). *Proc. Natl. Acad. Sci. U.S.A.* **85**, 2623.

Gough, N. M., Williams, R. L., Hilton, D. J., Pease, S. Willson, T. A., Stahl, J., Gearing, D. P., Nicola, N. A., and Metcalf, D. (1989). *Reprod. Fertil. Dev.* **1**, 281.

Hibi, M., Murakami, M., Saito, M., Hirano, T., Taga, T., and Kishimoto, T. (1990). *Cell* **63**, 1149.

Hilton, D. J., Nicola, N. A., and Metcalf, D. (1988). *Proc. Natl. Acad. Sci. U.S.A.* **85**, 5971.

Hirano, T., Akira, S., Taga, T., and Kishimoto, T. (1990). *Immunol. Today* **11**, 443.

Metcalf, D., and Gearing, D. P. (1989a). *Proc. Natl. Acad. Sci. U.S.A.* **86**, 5948.

Metcalf, D., and Gearing, D. P. (1989b). *Leukemia* **3**, 847.

Metcalf, D., Hilton, D. J., and Nicola, N. A. (1988). *Leukemia* **2**, 216.

Metcalf, D., Nicola, N. A., and Gearing, D. P. (1990). *Blood* **76**, 50.

Moreau, J. F., Donaldson, D. D., Bennett, F., Witeck-Giannotti, J., Clark, S. C., and Wong, G. G. (1988). *Nature (London)* **336**, 690.

Mori, M., Yamaguchi, K., and Abe, K. (1989). *Biochem. Biophys. Res. Commun.* **160**, 1085.

Reid, I. R., Lowe, C., Cornish, J., Skinner, S. J. M., Hilton, D. J., Willson, T. A., Gearing, D. P., and Martin, T. J. (1990). *Endocrinology (Baltimore)* **126**, 1416.

Taga, T., Hibi, M., Hirata, Y., Yamasaki, K., Yasukawa, K., Matsuda, T., Hirano, T., and Kishimoto, T. (1989). *Cell* **58**, 573.

Williams, R. L., Hilton, D. J., Pease, S., Willson, T. A., Stewart, C. L., Gearing, D. P., Wagner, E. F., Metcalf, D., Nicola, N. A., and Gough, N. M. (1988). *Nature (London)* **336**, 684.

Yamamori, T., Fukuda, K., Aebersold, R., Korsching, S., Fan, M.-J., Hood, L. E., and Patterson, P. H. (1989). *Science* **246**, 1412.

Comparative Pathology of Recombinant Murine Interferon-γ in Mice and Recombinant Human Interferon-γ in Cynomolgus Monkeys

Timothy G. Terrell and James D. Green
Department of Safety Evaluation
Genentech, Inc.
South San Francisco, California 94080

I. INTRODUCTION

The interferons represent a family of cytokines that share the capacity to induce resistance to viral infection in cells, as well as having a variety of other antiproliferative and immunomodulatory effects on cell functions (Vilcek *et al.,* 1985). Three major types of interferons have been identified. Leukocyte interferon (IFN-α) is the product of stimulated leukocytes, and several distinct species of IFN-α have been identified (Goeddel *et al.,* 1981). Fibroblast interferon (IFN-β) is derived from stimulated fibroblasts and is antigentically and structurally similar to IFN-α. Immune interferon (IFN-γ), originally described as the product of mitogen-stimulated leukocytes (Wheelock, 1965), has several distinct structural and functional differences from IFN-β and IFN-α. IFN-γ is produced by T lymphocytes following antigen or mitogen stimulation, and therefore is a true lymphokine. In contrast to both IFN-β and IFN-α, it is not induced by viruses. The gene for human IFN-γ is located on chromosome 12 (Naylor *et al.,* 1983), whereas the genes for IFN-α and IFN-β are on chromosome 9 (Owerbach *et al.,* 1981). IFN-γ has very little sequence homology to IFN-α or IFN-β (Gray and Goeddel, 1982), and it binds to a distinct cell surface receptor (Branca and Baglioni, 1981), whereas IFN-α and IFN-β cross-react with a common receptor.

Despite the structural differences between IFN-γ and the other interferons, they do share many common biological properties (Vilcek *et al.,* 1985), although IFN-γ has a generally broader range of activities than either IFN-α or IFN-β. The principal biological activities of IFN-γ are listed in Table I. Many cells and tissues are responsive to IFN-γ, suggesting that IFN-γ receptors are probably ubiquitous. The induction of cellular resistance to virus infection is the most characteristic feature of all interferons. Induction of protein synthesis is required for this antiviral activity, and the enzyme $2'5,'$-oligoadenylate synthetase is the best characterized of these proteins. Another activity shared by all of the interferons is the capacity to inhibit growth of many different cell types in culture. IFN-γ functions as an immunoregulatory protein as a result of its activities on lymphocytes and macrophages. Some of its immunoregulatory functions, such as induction of cytotoxic T lymphocytes, stimulation of natural killer (NK) cell activity, and induction of expression of major histocompatibility class I antigens (HLA-A, -B, and -C; H-2), are shared by the other interferons. IFN-γ also increases the synthesis and expression of major histocompatibility class II antigens (HLA-DR or Ia). The principal macrophage-activating factor (MAF) produced by

Table I. Principal Biological Activities of Interferon-γ[a]

Induction of resistance to viral infection
Inhibition of cell growth
Induction of cytotoxic T lymphocytes
Stimulation of NK cell activity
Induction of MHC class I and class II antigens
Inhibition of collagen synthesis
Activation of macrophages
Regulation of neutrophil migration
Induction of IL-2 receptors
Induction of Fc receptors
Stimulation of IL-1 and IL-2 synthesis
IL-4 antagonist
Cytokine synergy
Increased antibody production

[a] Modified from Vilcek *et al.* (1985).

normal T lymphocytes has been shown to be IFN-γ (Schreiber and Celada, 1985). It induces the expression of the IL-2 receptor on lymphocytes and the Fc receptor on marcophages. IFN-γ is also a potent inducer of IL-2 synthesis, an observation that is of interest because IL-2 is a major regulator of IFN-γ production (Farrar *et al.,* 1981). Stimulation of IL-1 production by IFN-γ (Haq *et al.,* 1985) is also consistent with its function as a macrophage-activating factor. IL-1 also induces its own gene expression, and IFN-γ down-regulates the synthesis of IL-1-induced IL-1 production (Ghezzi and Dinarello, 1988).

A high degree of interspecies homology exists at both the DNA and protein levels for many of the cytokines, which allows for testing of the efficacy and toxicity of the molecules in experimental animals (Remick and Kunkel, 1989). The biological activity of the interferons is, however, very species restricted. Although, both human IFN-α and IFN-β have been shown to exhibit some antiviral activity across species (Stewart, 1979), IFN-γ is very species specific (Gray and Goeddel, 1983) and has the most restricted host range activity of the interferons. Human IFN-γ is active on human cells and to a lesser extent on nonhuman primate cells, but not on cells of other mammalian species, such as the mouse and rat (Adolf, 1985). The advent of recombinant DNA technology has allowed for the preparation of sufficient quantities of purified proteins for *in vivo* experimentation. Both human and murine IFN-γ complementary DNAs have been cloned and expressed in cell systems (Gray and Goeddel, 1983; Gray *et al.,* 1982). The structure of murine IFN-γ cDNA has 64% nucleotide homology with human IFN-γ cDNA; however, the protein sequences of murine IFN-γ and human IFN-γ have only 40% homology (Gray and Goeddel, 1983; Dijkema *et al.,* 1985). This low homology of the proteins may explain the strict species specificity of IFN-γ.

One of the concerns in the toxicity testing of recombinant human IFN-γ (rHuIFN-γ) is that the species generally used for safety assessment may be of limited value due to the species specificity of the molecules. The preclinical toxicity studies with recombinant human IFN-α were generally not predictive of the treatment-related adverse effects observed in clinical trials with that molecule (Trown *et al.,* 1986). These studies were further complicated by the development of neutralizing antibodies to the human IFN-α, which may also have affected the toxicity of the proteins in the animals species studied. Often, the adverse effects seen in toxicity studies with cytokines and growth factors are exaggerated pharmacological effects of the molecules, and therefore can only be studied in a responsive species (Teelmann *et al.,* 1986; Hayes, 1990). More predictive toxicology results might be possible if the homologous IFN-γ is tested in each species. In this review, we will discuss the data obtained from a series of toxicity studies with rHuIFN-γ in a variety of species, and compare those findings with data from studies with recombinant murine IFN-γ (rMuIFN-γ) in the mouse.

II. EXPERIMENTAL FINDINGS

A. Acute Toxicity and Irritation Studies

A series of acute parenteral toxicity studies and parenteral and topical irritation studies of rHuIFN-γ were conducted in several species (Table II). In general, these studies were remarkable only in the absence of findings. Acute single-dose intravenous toxicity studies with rHuIFN-γ were performed in rats, marmosets, and squirrel monkeys. Human IFN-γ has not been shown to have biological activity in these species. In these studies a single dose of up to 10 mg/kg for the rat, 10 mg/animal (28 mg/kg) for the marmoset, and 5 mg/kg for the squirrel monkey was followed by a 14-day observation period. Standard clinical observations, body weight, body temperature, hematology, and serum chemistry determinations and necropsy evaluations were performed at the end of the observation period and selected tissues were examined histopathologically. No evidence of treatment-related toxicity was observed in any animal model tested. In another study, cynomolgus monkeys (*Macaca fascicularis*) were treated with escalating intravenous or subcutaneous doses of rHuIFN-γ at 4- to 5-day intervals (dose levels of 1.5, 15, 150, and 1500 μg/kg). No effects on body temperature, heart rate, blood pressure, or electrocardiograms were observed following dosing, and there was no evidence of antibodies to rHuIFN-γ on day 22.

The rHuIFN-γ formulation showed no evidence of irritative potential when tested in rabbits by a variety of routes of exposure, including intramuscular, subcutaneous, intraarterial, intravaginal, or ocular, or in squirrel mon-

Table II. Nonclinical Toxicology Studies with IFN-γ

Acute toxicity studies with rHuIFN-γ
  Rat, marmoset, squirrel monkey, and cynomolgus monkey; intravenous and subcutaneous
Subchronic toxicity studies with rHuIFN-γ
  Rat and cynomolgus monkey; intravenous and subcutaneous—10 days to 13 weeks
Developmental and reproductive toxicology with rHuIFN-γ
  Rat—segments I and II
  Rabbit—segment II
  Cynomolgus monkey—segments I and II
Special studies with rHuIFN-γ
  Irritation and tolerance—rabbit and squirrel monkey; intramuscular, intravenous, intraarterial,
    intravaginal, and ocular
  Guinea pig maximization
  In vitro hemolysis and mutation
Studies with rMuIFN-γ
  Subchronic toxicity in the mouse
  Segment II reproductive study in the mouse

---

keys by the intramuscular route. In addition, it did not demonstrate sensitization potential in the guinea pig maximization test.

B. Multidose Toxicity Studies with rHuIFN-γ

Multidose subchronic toxicity studies were conducted with rHuIFN-γ in rats and cynomolgus monkeys.

1. Subchronic Toxicity of rHuIFN-γ in the Rat

Subchronic toxicity studies of 3 months duration were conducted in rats with daily intravenous or intramuscular dosing. With the exception of the route of administration, the two studies were identical in design. Male and female rats received daily treatments with rHuIFN-γ at doses of 75, 250, or 750 μg/kg for 13 weeks, and a subset of animals, each in the control and high-dose groups, was allowed a 6-week treatment-free recovery period. The parameters evaluated included standard clinical observations, body weight, body temperature, food consumption, water intake, ophthalmologic findings, heart rate, hematology, clinical serum chemistry, urinalysis, gross pathology, organ weights, and microscopic pathology from a comprehensive list of tissues. Bone marrow smears were evaluated from animals in the control and high-dose groups. There were no remarkable clinical, hematology, or clinical chemistry changes noted in either study. No treatment-related gross or histopathological changes were observed at any dose. In the intravenous study, an increase in the number of plasma cells was observed in the bone marrow of animals treated with 750 μg/kg/day at the end of the treatment period. This change was interpreted as a manifestation of the immune response mounted against the rHuIFN-γ, and was not evident after the recovery period.

2. Subchronic Toxicity of rHuIFN-γ in the Cynomolgus Monkey

Two subchronic studies were conducted in cynomolgus monkeys. In one, monkeys were treated with rHuIFN-γ in a formulation containing 1% human serum albumin (HSA) by daily intravenous injections for 28 days at doses of 0.015, 0.15, and 1.5 mg/kg/day, which correlated with specific activity of 6×10^5, 6×10^6, and 6×10^7 U of rHuIFN-γ, respectively. The parameters evaluated were similar to those for the rodent studies with the addition of electrocardiograms. A dose-dependent increase in body temperature measured at 3 to 6 hr after treatment was observed during the first 2 weeks of treatment. Four animals, including all three males, in the 1.5-mg/kg dose group died between study days 19 and 25. Evidence of decreased hematopoietic function was observed in animals receiving doses of 0.15 or 1.5 mg/kg/day (Table III). This effect was observed for myeloid and ery-

Table III. Mean Hematologic Values in Cynomolgus Monkeys Treated with rHuIFN-γ Intravenously for 28 Days[a]

Parameter/dose (mg/kg/day)	Males			Females		
	Predose	Week 2	Week 4	Predose	Week 2	Week 4
Erythrocytes ($10^6/\mu$l)						
Control	6.49 (0.55)	6.50 (0.36)	6.47 (0.65)	5.76 (0.67)	5.66 (0.49)	5.81 (0.05)
0.015	6.56 (0.13)	6.42 (0.26)	6.55 (0.87)	6.41 (0.27)	6.06 (0.30)	5.84 (0.45)
0.15	6.31 (0.34)	5.80 (0.52)	5.26 (0.89)	6.57 (1.57)	6.03 (0.46)	5.12 (1.12)
1.5	6.29 (0.67)	4.92(0.46)**[b]	—[c]	6.26 (0.79)	5.74 (0.45)	5.62 (0.12)
Hematocrit (%)						
Control	39.5 (2.5)	39.3 (1.6)	38.4 (2.6)	37.0 (2.9)	35.8 (2.0)	35.0 (0.4)
0.015	40.5 (2.5)	38.6 (2.4)	39.2 (4.1)	39.8 (3.0)	36.6 (1.3)	35.0 (2.0)
0.15	40.9 (1.8)	36.6 (2.5)	33.7 (4.4)	39.2 (6.8)	35.3 (6.8)	30.2 (5.0)
1.5	39.0 (3.0)	30.5 (3.3)*	—	37.5 (3.0)	33.2 (3.0)	33.0 (0.7)*
Hemoglobin (g/dl)						
Control	12.3 (0.9)	12.2 (0.6)	11.8 (0.9)	10.8 (0.8)	10.6 (0.2)	10.2 (0.1)
0.015	12.3 (0.6)	12.1 (0.9)	12.1 (1.3)	12.0 (0.6)	11.1 (0.5)	10.7 (0.8)
0.15	12.3 (0.6)	11.3 (0.7)	9.8 (1.1)	11.4 (2.6)	10.2 (0.4)	8.8 (1.6)
1.5	12.0 (0.9)	9.3 (0.9)*	—	10.9 (0.7)	9.6 (0.2)**	9.3 (0.4)*

WBC ($10^3/\mu$l)						
Control	14.5 (5.7)	14.5 (5.1)	12.0 (4.5)	8.5 (2.1)	9.9 (2.8)	9.0 (2.4)
0.015	7.7 (0.7)	5.3 (0.4)	6.2 (1.5)	7.8 (2.7)	6.0 (1.6)	3.8 (1.7)
0.15	7.5 (1.4)	5.2 (2.8)	3.4 (0.7)	6.6 (0.7)	4.8 (1.3)	5.9 (3.8)
1.5	8.9 (2.0)	2.3 (0.4)	—	9.6 (1.4)	3.7 (0.7)*	5.1 (1.0)
Platelets ($10^3/\mu$l)						
Control	230.0 (62.9)	287.6 (35.7)	240.0 (25.5)	176.6 (44.0)	191.0 (21.0)	137.0 (7.5)
0.015	205.3 (28.8)	191.3 (44.7)*	177.3 (38.0)	253.3 (30.8)	223.3 (24.3)	151.0 (41.5)
0.15	182.3 (13.6)	156.6 (34.6)*	153.0 (12.0)**	228.3 (71.9)	133.6 (42.7)	157.0 (67.1)
1.5	184.3 (43.0)	121.0 (29.5)**	—	198.3 (41.9)	179.3 (34.2)	186.5 (21.9)*

[a] Hematology parameters measured on blood collected predose and during weeks 2 and 4; $N = 3$ animals/sex, except for the 4-week 1.5-mg/kg/day female group that had only two survivors. No treatment-related changes were observed for reticulocyte counts, fibrinogen, or prothrombin time. Changes in WBCs were primarily due to decreased numbers of neutrophils. Standard deviations shown in parentheses.

[b] Statistically significant when compared to controls of same sex using the Student's t test. *, $p < 0.05$; **, $p < 0.01$.

[c] No surviving males in the 1.5-mg/kg/day group at 4 weeks.

throid components and was characterized by decreased erythrocyte counts, hemoglobin, and hematocrit; decreased leukocyte counts primarily due to marked neutropenia; and thrombocytopenia. Decreased cellularity with a reduction in the myeloid to erythroid (M:E) ratio was observed in the bone marrow. Serum chemistry changes included increased aspartate amino-transferase (AST), lactic dehydrogenase (LDH), and triglyceride values in animals receiving doses of 0.15 or 1.5 mg/kg/day (Table IV). A marginal decrease in albumin was also observed in the high-dose females. Changes in clinical pathology parameters were more severe and occurred earlier in animals receiving the 1.5-mg/kg dose compared to those receiving 0.15 mg/kg.

Histopathological changes were primarily observed in animals receiving doses of 0.15 mg/kg or greater, with dose-dependent increases in incidence and severity (Table V). Thymic atrophy characterized by depletion of lymphocytes from the cortex of the thymus correlated with decreased organ weights for thymus at necropsy and was observed in all high-dose animals. Lymphoid depletion was also observed in splenic follicles and mesenteric lymph nodes, and decreased myeloid cellularity was present in the bone marrow. Hepatic changes were characterized by diffuse slight to moderate hepatocellular atrophy with dilatation of sinusoidal spaces, and multifocal areas of slight hepatocellular degeneration in some animals. Diffuse slight to moderate hypertrophy of reticuloendothelial cells lining the hepatic sinusoids, suggestive of activation of the reticuloendothelial system (RES), was present in all high-dose animals. Interferon-γ is a macrophage-activating factor, and the RE cell hyperplasia is consistent with a direct effect of the rHuIFN-γ that was administered. Several of the animals that died had mucosal ulcerations in the gastrointestinal tract, particularly the esophagus, stomach, colon, cecum, and rectum. Similar changes were not observed in animals that survived the treatment. Other changes that were observed in some animals that died included focal fibrosis and/or degeneration in the heart and lung. The occurrence of this change was sporadic, and it may represent a coincidental lesion rather than a treatment effect. Decreased spermatogenesis was present in the testes of males from each of the treatment groups, but not in control males.

Four of eight animals in the mid- and high-dose groups developed high titers of neutralizing antibody to the rHuIFN-γ. There did not appear to be any correlation between the increased antibody formation and the subsequent condition of the test animals.

In a second study, cynomolgus monkeys were treated with rHuIFN-γ in a formulation containing 1% human serum albumin (HSA) by daily intramuscular injections for 90 days. Based on the results of the previous 28-day study, the highest dose used in this study was 0.15 mg/kg/day, which correlated with specific activity of 6×10^6 U of rHuIFN-γ. Low- and mid-dose levels were 0.0015 and 0.015 mg/kg/day, which correlated with specific

Table IV. Mean Serum Chemistry Values in Cynomolgus Monkeys Treated with rHuIFN-γ Intravenously for 28 days[a]

Parameter/dose (mg/kg/day)	Males			Females		
	Predose	Week 2	Week 4	Predose	Week 2	Week 4
AST (IU/liter)						
Control	13.1 (4.6)	14.7 (7.0)	13.6 (6.3)	17.6 (5.5)	22.8 (6.4)	48.3 (31.5)
0.015	15.4 (6.3)	14.6 (1.5)	29.3 (26.7)	17.0 (9.9)	15.8 (6.3)	17.3 (2.6)
0.15	12.8 (6.3)	18.7 (11.3)	42.0 (31.1)	17.7 (2.7)	25.4 (10.7)	184.7 (258.3)
1.5	15.2 (3.0)	86.3 (67.2)	—[b]	12.9 (4.8)	21.1 (3.0)	101.8 (94.1)
LDH (IU/liter)						
Control	578.3 (93.0)	734.8 (100.2)	621.0 (137.3)	740.5 (338.3)	616.3 (246.5)	701.2 (149.4)
0.015	734.1 (364.9)	652.2 (122.9)	975.1 (573.5)	615.3 (125.9)	622.2 (215.2)	705.5 (138.6)
0.15	526.1 (45.1)	849.6 (121.9)	2570.0 (2791.7)	584.3 (21.2)	966.8 (326.8)	3956.2 (4941.0)
1.5	604.5 (118.0)	3353.0 (1595.3)	—	624.2 (136.3)	966.8 (132.9)	2424.7 (984.9)
Triglycerides (mg/dl)						
Control	65.9 (33.0)	71.8 (32.8)	63.5 (18.5)	69.9 (35.5)	67.3 (15.2)	97.9 (26.4)
0.015	82.5 (18.7)	76.3 (18.9)	101.0 (42.3)	82.8 (17.3)	91.7 (12.0)	105.3 (27.4)
0.15	76.8 (25.7)	101.7 (41.0)	151.3 (102.5)	89.2 (37.0)	127.7 (33.1)[*c]	345.7 (202.5)
1.5	58.2 (7.7)	247.6 (183.7)	—	74.3 (28.0)	123.2 (42.9)	278.7 (121.8)
Albumin (g/dl)						
Control	3.5 (0.2)	3.4 (0.2)	3.5 (0.2)	3.3 (0.0)	3.3 (0.05)	3.4 (0.05)
0.015	3.4 (0.2)	3.6 (0.1)	3.7 (0.1)	3.5 (0.1)	3.6 (0.2)	3.6 (0.05)*
0.15	3.4 (0.05)	3.5 (0.1)	3.2 (0.6)	3.3 (0.05)	3.4 (0.05)	3.1 (0.2)
1.5	3.3 (0.1)	3.2 (0.05)	—	3.2 (0.1)	3.4 (0.2)	2.9 (0.07)**

[a] Serum chemistry parameters measured on blood collected predose and during weeks 2 and 4; $N = 3$ animals/sex, except for the 4-week 1.5-mg/kg/day female group that had only two survivors. No treatment-related changes were observed for alanine aminotransferase, alkaline phosphatase, blood urea nitrogen, total cholesterol, total protein, A:G ratio, cholinesterase, calcium, creatinine, total bilirubin, phosphate, glucose, amylase, sodium, potassium, or chloride. Standard deviations shown in parentheses.

[b] No surviving males in the 1.5-mg/kg/day group at 4 weeks.

[c] Statistically significant when compared to controls of same sex using the Student's t test. *, $p < 0.05$; **, $p < 0.01$.

Table V. Incidence and Severity of Selected Histopathological Lesions in Cynomolgus Monkeys Treated with rHuIFN-γ Intravenously for 28 Days

Tissue/Lesion	Dose (mg/kg/day)			
	Control	0.015	0.15	1.5
Thymus				
Lymphoid depletion	−[a]	−	+ (1/6)[b]	++ (6/6)
Spleen				
Lymphoid depletion follicular	−	−	++ (2/6)	++ (6/6)
Mesenteric lymph node				
Lymphoid depletion	−	−	+ (2/6)	+ (3/6)
Bone marrow				
Decreased cellularity, myeloid	−	−	+ (3/6)	++ (5/6)
Testes				
Seminiferous tubular atrophy	−	+ (1/3)	+ (1/3)	++ (2/3)
Hypospermatogenesis	−	++ (2/3)	++ (1/3)	++ (2/3)
Liver				
Hepatocellular atrophy	−	−	+ (1/6)	++ (5/6)
Hepatocellular degeneration	−	−	++ (1/6)	++ (2/6)
Reticuloendothelial cell hypertrophy	−	−	+ (1/6)	++ (6/6)
Esophagus				
Mucosal ulceration	−	−	−	++[c] (2/6)
Stomach				
Mucosal ulceration	−	−	−	+[c] (2/6)
Large intestine				
Mucosal ulceration	−	−	−	++[c] (3/6)

[a] Lesion severity grades: −, not present; +, slight; ++, moderate; +++, severe.

[b] Number of animals with lesion present/number of animals examined.

[c] Mucosal ulceration was only observed in those animals that died during the study.

activity of 6×10^4 and 6×10^5 U of rHuIFN-γ, respectively. At the termination of the treatment period, three animals/sex/group were euthanized and necropsied. Two animals of each sex from the control and high-dose groups were maintained for an additional treatment-free recovery period of 5 weeks. The parameters evaluated were similar to the 28-day study. Clinical pathology parameters were evaluated prior to initiation of dosing, after 4 weeks of treatment, at the end of the treatment period and after the recovery period.

Changes that were observed were similar to some of those in the 28-day study; however, they were less striking and had a lower incidence. Body temperatures were elevated at doses of 0.015 mg/kg and above. Clinical pathology parameters revealed a slight depression of hematologic values, including erythrocyte count, hematocrit, and hemoglobin. These changes were only evident at the high-dose level at the 5-week interval. Neutropenia and thrombocytopenia were also observed at both the 5-week interval and at termination of the treatment, but were reversed after the 5-week recovery period. Histopathological evaluation of bone marrow at termination of the treatment period revealed an increase in cellularity of myeloid precursors, suggesting a hyperplastic change rather than depression of bone marrow function at that time. Serum chemistry changes included increased AST, triglycerides, LDH, and creatine phosphokinase, and decreased total cholesterol. Albumin was marginally decreased, and total protein was increased, primarily due to increased globulin content. Antibody titers against rHuIFN-γ were detected in all groups after 5 weeks. The increased globulin may reflect that antibody response against rHuIFN-γ. The neutralizing antibody response to the rHuIFN-γ may have resulted in an amelioration of many of the effects of the treatment, including the effects on body temperature and hematology parameters.

Diffuse slight to moderate RE cell hypertrophy and hyperplasia were observed in the liver (Fig. 1) and spleen of animals treated with doses of 0.015 mg/kg and above (Table VI). Bone marrow of high-dose animals had marked hyperplasia of myeloid elements. Another lesion observed in a majority of the high-dose animals was a proliferative glomerulitis characterized by an increase in mesangial matrix with proliferation of the glomerular epithelium (Fig. 2). Morphologically, the lesion resembled an immune complex glomerulitis; however, electron microscopsy failed to demonstrate immune deposits in the basement membrane. It is possible that the lesion was a result of the antibody response against the rHuIFN-γ. Other lesions observed in the 4-week study were not present in animals in this study, including thymic and lymphoid atrophy, gastrointestinal ulceration, cardiomyopathy, and, especially, hypospermatogenesis, which was present in some males treated with 0.015 mg/kg in the 4-week study. All lesions, including the glomerulonephritis, showed evidence of reversal with cessation of treatment.

C. Subchronic Toxicity of rMuIFN-γ in the Mouse

Because rHuIFN-γ is not biologically active in the mouse, a toxicity study was conducted with recombinant murine IFN-γ in mice in an effort to

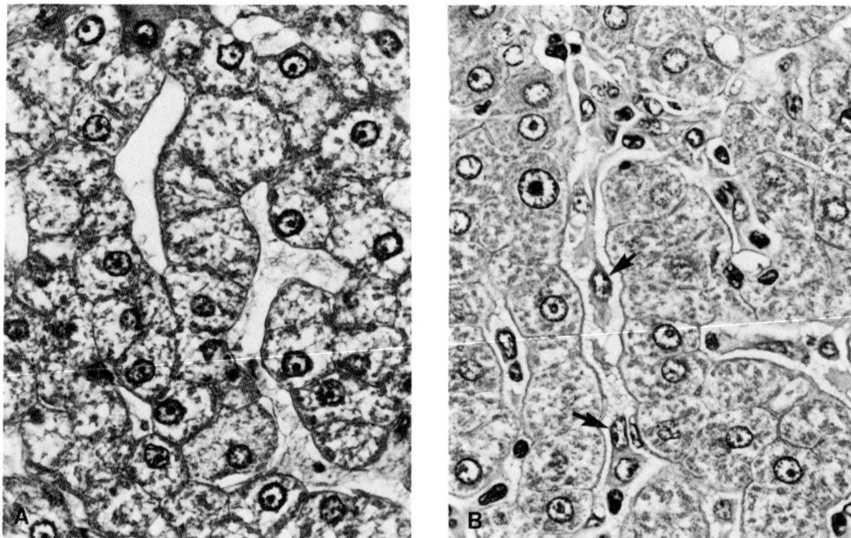

Fig. 1. (a) Normal liver from a control cynomolgus monkey. Hematoxylin and eosin (×800). (b) Liver from a cynomolgus monkey given 0.15 mg/kg/day rHuIFN-γ, intravenously, for 90 days. Marked hyperplasia and hypertrophy of reticuloendothelial cells lining the hepatic sinusoids. Hematoxylin and eosin (×800).

Table VI. Incidence and Severity of Histopathological Lesions in Cynomolgus Monkeys Treated with rHuIFN-γ Intravenously for 90 Days

	Dose (mg/kg/day)			
Tissue/lesion	Control	0.0015	0.015	0.15
Spleen				
Reticuloendothelial cell hypertrophy	$-^a$	−	++ (2/6)^b	++ (6/6)
Liver				
Reticuloendothelial cell hypertrophy	−	−	+ (4/6)	++ (5/6)
Kidney				
Glomerulonephritis	−	−	+ (1/6)	++ (5/6)
Bone marrow				
Increased hematopoietic cellularity	−	−	+ (1/6)	+ (2/6)

[a] Lesion severity grades: −, not present; +, slight; ++, moderate; +++, severe.
[b] Number of animals with lesion present/number of animals examined.

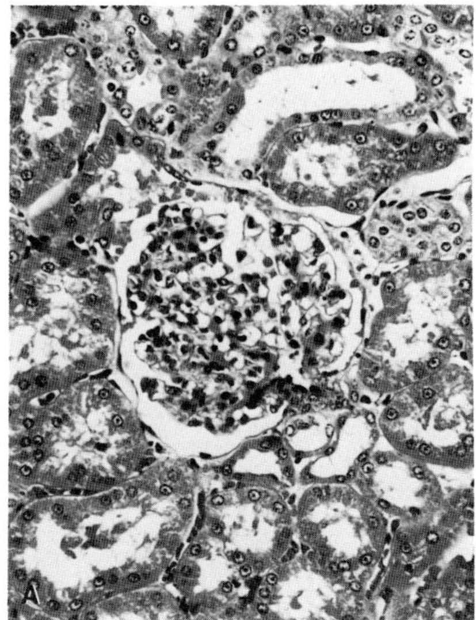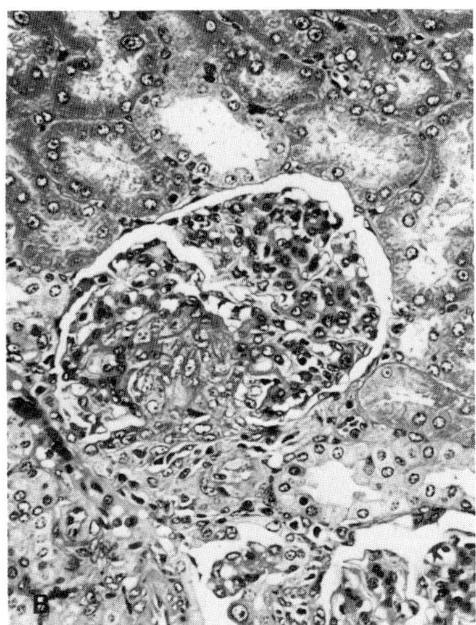

Fig. 2. (a) Normal kidney from a control cynomolgus monkey. Hematoxylin and eosin (×320). (b) Kidney from a cynomolgus monkey given 0.15 mg/kg/day rHuIFN-γ, intravenously, for 90 days. Glomerulonephritis with increased mesangial matrix with proliferation of glomerular epithelial cells. Hematoxylin and eosin (×320).

predict the potential toxicity of rHuIFN-γ in humans. The rMuIFN-γ was administered to male and female C3H/He mice by daily intramuscular injections for 28 days at doses of 0.023, 0.23, and 2.32 mg/kg/day (equivalent to 10^5, 10^6, and 10^7 U/kg/day, respectively). The parameters evaluated included clinical observations, body weight, body temperature, food consumption, ophthalmologic findings, hematology, clinical serum chemistry, urinalysis, gross pathology, organ weights, and microscopic pathology from a comprehensive list of tissues, including bone marrow smears.

Suppression of body weight gain was observed at the high dose. No effect on body temperature was detected. There was no detectable antibody formation to the rMuIFN-γ in treated groups. A slight decrease in hematocrit and hemoglobin and the associated red cell parameters, but not erythrocyte counts, was observed at the high dose (Table VII). No effect on leukocyte counts was observed. Serum biochemistry evaluations revealed elevations in ALT, AST, ALP, LDH, and LAP at doses of 0.23 and 2.32 mg/kg/day (Table VIII). Blood glucose and cholesterol levels were decreased.

Gross pathology changes present in mice at the scheduled necropsy included liver and splenic enlargement with a dose-related increase in absolute and relative organ weights in the mice treated with rMuIFN-γ (Table IX). Thymus weights were decreased as compared to controls in mice treated at the high dose. Bilateral testicular atrophy was observed in many of

Table VII. Mean Hematologic Values in Mice Treated with rMuIFN-γ Intramuscularly for 28 Days[a]

Dose (mg/kg/day)	N	Erythrocytes ($10^6/\mu l$)	Hematocrit (%)	Hemoglobin (g/dl)	MCV (fl)	MCH (pg)	MCHC (%)	WBC ($10^3/\mu l$)
Males								
Control	10	8.58 (0.07)	48.5 (0.5)	14.5 (0.1)	56.5 (0.3)	16.8 (0.1)	29.8 (0.2)	2.5 (0.4)
Placebo	10	8.74 (0.06)	49.0 (0.4)	14.6 (0.1)	56.1 (0.2)	16.7 (0.1)	29.8 (0.2)	3.3 (0.3)
0.023	10	9.15 (0.12)*[b]	50.9 (0.7)	15.1 (0.2)*	55.8 (0.2)	16.5 (0.1)*	29.7 (0.1)	3.0 (0.4)
0.23	9	9.12 (0.20)*	49.8 (1.3)	14.7 (0.3)	54.6 (0.4)*	16.2 (0.1)*	29.6 (0.3)	3.2 (0.6)
2.32	10	8.54 (0.37)	44.6 (2.1)	12.9 (0.6)*	52.2 (0.6)*	15.1 (0.1)*	29.0 (0.1)*	2.6 (0.4)
Females								
Control	10	8.94 (0.09)	50.6 (0.4)	15.3 (0.2)	56.4 (0.2)	17.1 (0.1)	30.2 (0.2)	3.2 (0.3)
Placebo	10	8.60 (0.12)	49.5 (0.7)	14.9 (0.2)	56.2 (0.3)	16.9 (0.2)	30.0 (0.3)	3.2 (0.4)
0.023	9	8.97 (0.17)	50.0 (1.0)	15.0 (0.3)	55.7 (0.2)*	16.7 (0.1)*	30.0 (0.3)	2.9 (0.2)
0.23	10	9.11 (0.11)	50.7 (0.5)	14.8 (0.1)*	55.6 (0.4)	16.2 (0.1)*	29.1 (0.1)*	4.1 (1.3)
2.32	9	8.87 (0.10)	45.7 (0.4)*	13.2 (0.2)*	51.7 (0.6)*	14.9 (0.1)*	28.9 (0.2)*	2.3 (0.4)

[a] Hematology parameters measured on blood collected from mice 24 hr after the last treatment; N = number of mice evaluated. No treatment-related changes were observed for reticulocytes, platelets, or differential counts for lymphocytes, neutrophils, eosinophils, monocytes, or basophils. Standard error of the mean shown in parentheses.

[b] Statistically significant when compared to controls of same sex using the Student's t test. *, $p < 0.05$; **, $p < 0.01$.

Table VIII. Mean Serum Chemistry Values in Mice Treated with rMuIFN-γ Intramuscularly for 28 Days[a]

Dose (mg/kg/day)	N	ALT (IU/liter)	AST (IU/liter)	ALP (K.A.U.)[c]	LAP (IU/liter)	LDH (IU/liter)	Glucose (mg/dl)	Cholesterol (mg/dl)
Males								
Control	10	24 (3)	64 (4)	11.0 (0.4)	37 (2)	1183 (155)	200 (7)	140 (3)
Placebo	10	20 (1)	62 (3)	10.0 (0.5)	41 (1)	1106 (167)	200 (9)	142 (3)
0.023	10	23 (1)	61 (4)	11.7 (0.3)	47 (1)*	872 (71)	215 (9)	146 (3)
0.23	9	42 (2)*[b]	96 (4)*	15.8 (0.5)*	65 (1)*	1052 (83)	168 (9)*	121 (3)*
2.32	10	96 (5)*	219 (33)*	13.0 (0.6)*	78 (2)*	1971 (171)*	127 (7)*	85 (4)*
Females								
Control	9	25 (1)	77 (5)	16.4 (0.2)	36 (2)	963 (101)	184 (4)	113 (3)
Placebo	10	23 (1)	72 (3)	14.6 (0.5)*	36 (1)	1024 (112)	185 (5)	111 (4)
0.023	9	28 (1)	83 (5)	16.6 (0.6)	46 (1)*	898 (134)	188 (6)	95 (5)*
0.23	10	40 (1)*	108 (4)*	25.4 (0.9)*	65 (1)*	1009 (72)	182 (6)	89 (2)*
2.32	9	96 (1)*	197 (5)*	19.9 (0.8)*	85 (1)*	1747 (50)*	149 (7)*	83 (1)*

[a] Clinical chemistry analysis performed on blood collected from mice 24 hr after the last treatment; N = number of mice evaluated. ALT, Alanine aminotransferase; AST, aspartate aminotransferase; ALP, alkaline phosphatase; LDH, lactate dehydrogenase; LAP, leucine aminopeptidase. No treatment-related changes were observed for cholinesterase, total bilirubin, creatine phosphokinase, urea nitrogen, uric acid, total protein, albumin, inorganic phosphorus, triglyceride, sodium, potassium, chloride, or calcium. Standard error of the mean shown in parentheses.

[b] Statistically significant when compared to controls of same sex using the Student's t test. *, $p < 0.05$; **, $p < 0.01$.

[c] K.A.U., King–Armstrong units.

Table IX. Mean Organ Weight Values for Mice Treated with rMuIFN-γ Intramuscularly for 28 Days[a]

Dose (mg/kg/day)	N	Liver	Spleen	Thymus	Testis
Males					
Control	10	1.13 (0.02)	0.075 (0.001)	0.037 (0.003)	0.17 (0.00)
Placebo	10	1.17 (0.03)	0.083 (0.001)	0.032 (0.002)	0.17 (0.00)
0.023	10	1.22 (0.03)*[b]	0.105 (0.002)*	0.039 (0.003)	0.17 (0.00)
0.23	9	1.31 (0.02)*	0.159 (0.004)*	0.037 (0.004)	0.18 (0.00)
2.32	10	1.43 (0.07)*	0.219 (0.012)*	0.025 (0.002)*	0.07 (0.01)*
Females					
Control	10	1.08 (0.03)	0.095 (0.003)	0.041 (0.001)	—
Placebo	10	1.08 (0.03)	0.101 (0.005)	0.044 (0.001)	—
0.023	9	1.14 (0.03)	0.126 (0.004)*	0.044 (0.002)	—
0.23	10	1.24 (0.02)*	0.175 (0.010)*	0.039 (0.004)	—
2.32	9	1.43 (0.05)*	0.237 (0.029)*	0.032 (0.002)*	—

[a] Mean organ weights in grams for animals necropsied after 28 days of treatment. There were no treatment-related changes in weights for kidney, heart, lung, and brain. Standard error of the mean shown in parentheses.

[b] Statistically significant when compared to controls of same sex using the Student's t test. *, $p < 0.05$; **, $p < 0.01$.

the high-dose group males, as was a marked decrease in mean weight of the testes.

Histopathological lesions caused by the treatment were present in a large number of organs (Table X). Diffuse hypertrophy of reticuloendothelial cells lining the hepatic sinusoids (Fig. 3) and in the red pulp of the spleen and of reticulum cells in the bond marrow, suggestive of activation of the RES, was present in rMuIFN-γ-treated mice. This change was present in the majority of mice that were treated with 0.23 or 2.32 mg/kg/day. Increased prominence of sinusoidal macrophages in the adrenal gland, and infiltration of foamy macrophages into alveolar septae of the lungs, were also consistent with widespread activation of the RES. Stimulation of hematopoietic activity was evident by the increased numbers of immature hematopoietic precursor cells in the bone marrow (Fig. 4) and increased extramedullary hematopoiesis (erythroid and granulocytic) in the spleen. Thymic atrophy, characterized by depletion of lymphocytes from the cortex of the thymus, and lymphoid depletion in splenic follicles and mesenteric lymph nodes were observed in some high-dose mice.

All high-dose males had marked atrophy of the seminiferous tubules of the testes with diffuse hypospermatogenesis (Fig. 5); however, similar changes were not observed at lower doses. The testicular atrophy was accompanied by a decreased presence of sperm in the tubules of the epididymides, and accumulation of cellular debris from degenerating spermatozoa. A slight increase in evidence of atretric follicles was observed in females of the mid- and high-dose groups, with accompaning atrophy of the uterus in high-dose females.

Table X. Incidence and Severity of Histopathological Lesions in Mice Treated with rMuIFN-γ Intramuscularly for
28 Days

Tissue/Lesion	Dose (mg/kg/day)				
	Control	Placebo	0.023	0.23	2.32
Thymus					
Lymphoid depletion	−[a]	−	NE[b]	−	+ (2/20)[c]
Spleen					
Lymphoid depletion	−	−	−	−	+ (1/20)
Increased extramedullary hematopoiesis	−	−	−	+ (11/19)	++ (19/20)
Reticuloendothelial cell hypertrophy	−	−	−	+ (4/19)	++ (16/19)
Mesenteric lymph node					
Lymphoid depletion	−	+ (1/19)	−	+ (3/19)	++ (14/18)
Bone Marrow					
Increased cellularity, hematopoietic	−	+ (1/20)	+ (5/20)	+ (7/20)	++ (19/19)
Reticulum cell hypertrophy	−	−	−	−	++ (19/19)
Testes					
Hypospermatogensis	−	−	−	−	++ (10/10)
Liver					
Hepatocellular atrophy	−	−	−	−	+ (1/19)
Reticuloendothelial cell hypertrophy	−	−	+ (2/9)	++ (19/19)	++ (19/19)
Lung					
Foamy cell infiltration, alveolar septae	−	−	−	−	+ (9/20)
Heart					
Degeneration of cardiomyofiber	−	−	−	+ (3/19)	++ (19/19)
Histiocyte infiltration	+ (2/20)	+ (3/20)	−	+ (5/20)	++ (19/19)
Mineralization	+ (6/20)	+ (10/20)	+ (4/19)	+ (7/20)	++ (19/20)
Stomach					
Undifferentiated epithelium, hypercellularity	−	+ (1/20)	−	−	+ (17/19)
Histiocytic infiltration	+ (5/20)	+ (5/20)	+ (9/19)	+ (13/19)	+ (14/19)
Small intestine					
Increased mitotic activity, crypt	−	−	−	+ (5/18)	++ (17/18)

(Continued)

Table X. (*Continued*)

Tissue/Lesion	Dose (mg/kg/day)				
	Control	Placebo	0.023	0.23	2.32
Histiocytic infiltration, lamina propria	−	−	+ (1/19)	+ (18/18)	++ (17/18)
Colon					
Increased mitotic activity, crypt	−	−	+ (2/19)	+ (1/19)	+ (11/19)
Decreased epithelial mucous	−	−	+ (2/19)	+ (6/19)	++ (17/19)
Adrenal					
Atrophy of X zone	−	+ (1/19)	−	−	++ (19/19)
Hypertrophy, zona fasciculata	−	−	+ (2/20)	+ (7/19)	+ (8/19)
Hypertrophy, sinusoidal macrophages	−	−	−	+ (11/19)	+ (11/19)
Pituitary					
Atrophy of acidophils	−	−	−	+ (9/19)	++ (17/17)
Pancreas					
Nuclear hypertrophy, acinar cells	−	−	−	+ (15/20)	++ (18/19)
Salivary gland					
Acinar atrophy	−	−	−	+ (4/20)	++ (19/19)

[a] Lesion severity grades: −, not present; +, slight; ++, moderate; +++, severe.
[b] NE, Not examined.
[c] Number of animals with lesion present/number of animals examined.

A variety of morphlogical lesions were evident in the mucosal lining of the gastrointestinal tract, involving the stomach, duodenum, jejunum, and colon. In the stomach, there was hypertrophy of parietal cells, atrophy of chief cells, and a marked hypercellularity of undifferentiated epithelial cells in the neck of the gastric glands (Fig. 6). The proliferation of undifferentiated epithelium was a prominent change in the small and large intestine sections also. Diffuse infiltration of inflammatory cells into the lamina propria was observed in the stomach and small intestine. The infiltrate was composed of histiocytes and lymphocytes.

A mild cardiomyopathy characterized by areas of degeneration of myofibers and infiltration of histiocytes (Fig. 7) was observed in the majority of the animals in the high-dose group, and to a lesser extent in mid-dose animals. Cardiac mineralization, which is not an uncommon finding in female C3H/He mice, but is less frequently observed in males, was increased in

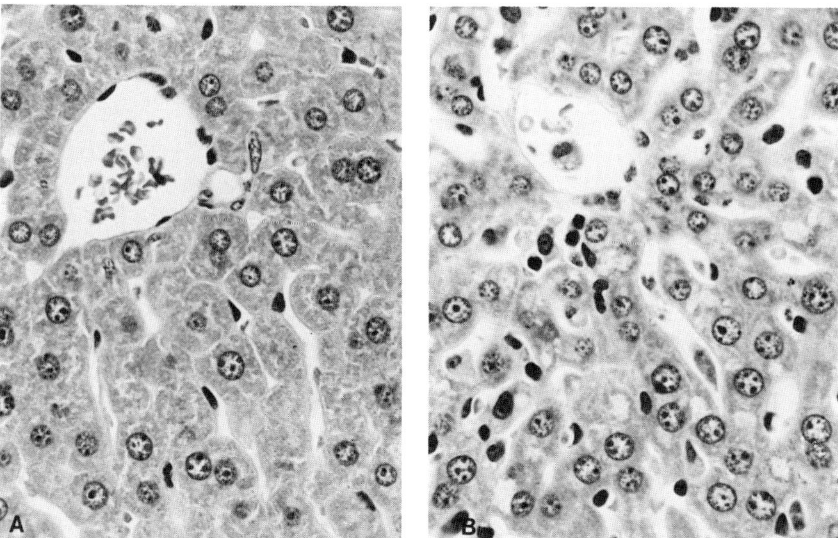

Fig. 3. (a) Normal liver from a control mouse. Hematoxylin and eosin (×800). (b) Liver from a mouse given 2.32 mg/kg/day rMuIFN-γ, intramuscularly, for 28 days. Marked hyperplasia and hypertrophy of reticuloendothelial cells lining the hepatic sinusoids with atrophy of hepatocytes. Hematoxylin and eosin (×800).

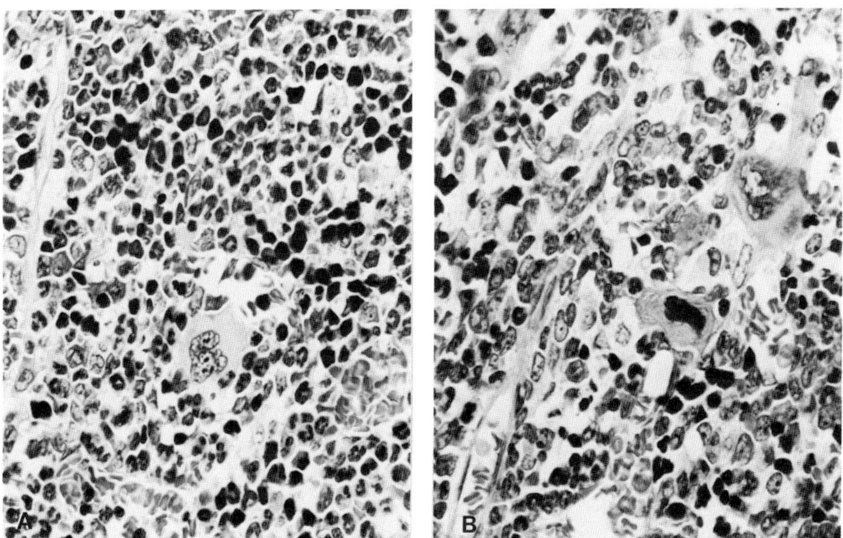

Fig. 4. (a) Normal bone marrow from a control mouse. Hematoxylin and eosin (×800). (b) Bone marrow from a mouse given 2.32 mg/kg/day rMuIFN-γ, intramuscularly, for 28 days. Depletion of mature granulocytes and proliferation of reticulum cells. Hematoxylin and eosin (×800).

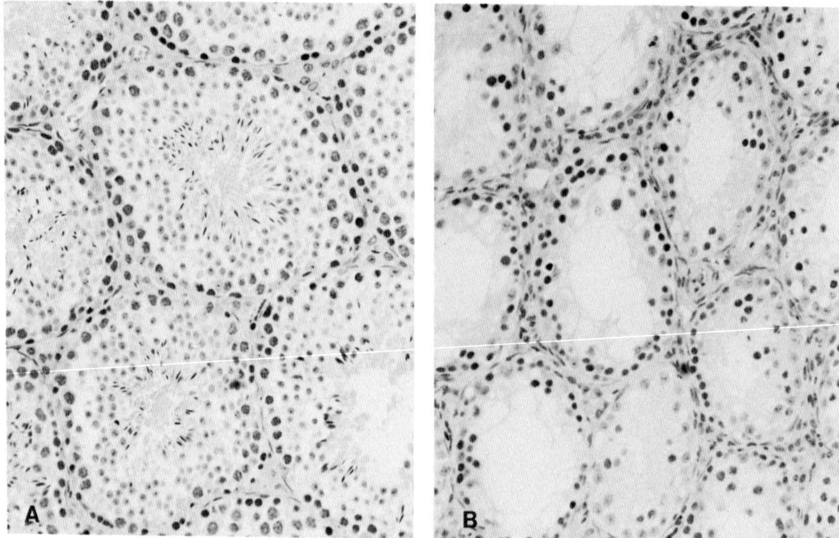

Fig. 5. (a) Normal testis from a control mouse. Hematoxylin and eosin (×320). (b) Testis from a mouse given 2.32 mg/kg/day rMuIFN-γ, intramuscularly, for 28 days. Hypospermatogenesis with atrophy of seminiferous tubules and vacuolation of Sertoli cells. Hematoxylin and eosin (×320).

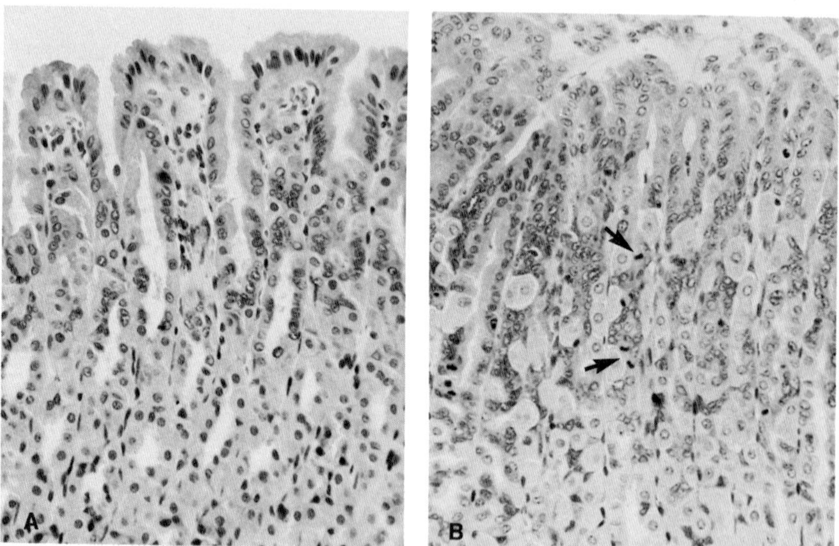

Fig. 6. (a) Normal stomach from a control mouse. Hematoxylin and eosin (×320). (b) Stomach from a mouse given 2.32 mg/kg/day rMuIFN-γ, intramuscularly, for 28 days. Increased mitotic activity (arrow) with hypercellularity of undifferentiated epithelial cells in the neck of the gland. Hematoxylin and eosin (×320).

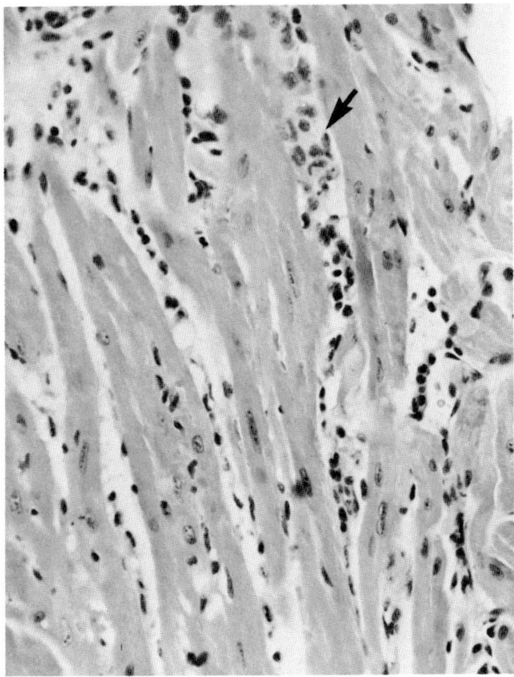

Fig. 7. Heart from a mouse given 2.32 mg/kg/day rMuIFN-γ, intramuscularly, for 28 days. Degeneration of myofibers with infiltration of histiocytes (arrow). Hematoxylin and eosin (×320).

incidence and severity at the high-dose level. Diffuse, mild infiltration of foamy histiocytic cells was observed in the alveolar septa of the lung of animals in the high-dose group (Fig. 8).

Atrophy of the X zone was observed in the adrenal glands of the high-dose males and females, and was accompanied by hypertrophy of the zona fasciculata in treated males. Atrophy of acidophils in the pars distalis of the pituitary gland was observed in high-dose males and females (Fig. 9). Other epithelial cell changes included acinar atrophy of the submaxillary salivary gland and nuclear hypertrophy with a decrease in content of zymogen granules in the acinar cells of the pancreas in males and females of the mid- and high-dose groups.

D. Reproductive and Developmental Toxicity Studies

1. Reproductive Studies with rHuIFN-γ in Rats

The effect of rHuIFN-γ on reproductive performance and fetal development was evaluated in male and female rats in segment I and segment II studies.

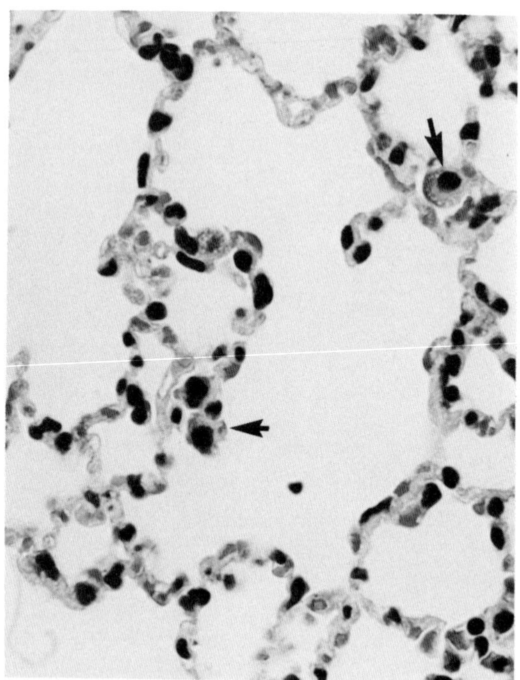

Fig. 8. Lung from a mouse given 2.32 mg/kg/day rMuIFN-γ, intramuscularly, for 28 days. Accumulation of foamy histiocytes (arrows) in the alveolar septa. Hematoxylin and eosin (×800).

Males received daily intravenous injections of 0.017, 0.09, or 0.43 mg/kg/day for 63 days prior to mating and 28 days after the start of mating; females were treated similarly for 14 days prior to mating, during the mating period, and until day 7 of gestation. Males were necropsied at the end of the treatment period and females were necropsied on day 20 of gestation and the reproductive tracts were removed for examination. Corpora lutea were counted on the ovaries, and uteri were examined for the number of implantation sites and viable and dead fetuses. Fetuses were examined for external abnormalities, and skeletal and visceral examinations were performed. Treatment of rats with rHuIFN-γ during the premating, mating, and early gestation had no effect on the reproductive performance of either sex or on fetal development.

The potential development toxicity of rHuIFN-γ was evaluated in pregnant rats treated with daily intravenous doses of 0.13, 0.4, and 1.3 mg/kg on days 7–16 of gestation. Dams were sacrificed on gestation day 22 and the reproductive tracts were removed and examined as described above. The treatment with rHuIFN-γ did not cause maternal toxicity, and rHuIFN-γ did

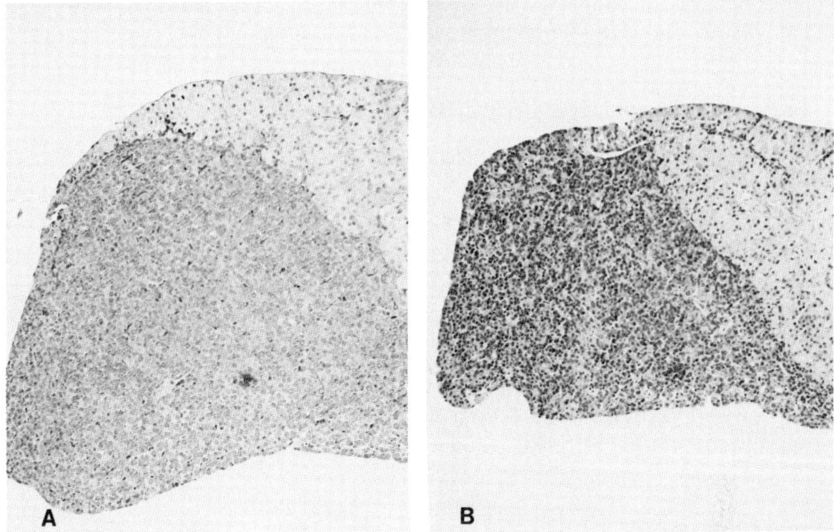

Fig. 9. (a) Normal pituitary from a control mouse. Hematoxylin and eosin (×80). (b) Pituitary from a mouse given 2.32 mg/kg/day rMuIFN-γ, intramuscularly, for 28 days. Atrophy of the pars distalis with decreased number of acidophil cells. Hematoxylin and eosin (×80).

not exhibit embryotoxic, fetotoxic, or teratogenic potential. In a second modified segment II study, pregnant rats were treated with daily i.v. doses of 0.022, 0.11, or 0.54 mg/kg on days 7–17 of gestation. Two-thirds of the dams were sacrificed on gestation day 20 and were examined, and the remaining dams were allowed to deliver. The offspring were evaluated for postnatal physical development, performance in behavioral tests, and reproductive function. No effects were observed on maternal of fetal indices or on postnatal development.

2. Reproductive Studies with rHuIFN-γ in Cynomolgus Monkeys

The potential reproductive toxicity of rHuIFN-γ was evaluated in a segment II study in cynomolgus monkeys (Lewandowski *et al.,* 1991). Females received daily subcutaneous injections of 0.003, 0.03, or 0.15 mg/kg from day 20 to day 80 of gestation. During treatment, females were monitored for clinical signs of toxicity and blood was collected periodically for analysis of hormone levels and antibody formation. The pregnancies were terminated by cesarean section on day 100 ± 1 of gestation, and fetuses were examined for external, visceral, and skeletal abnormalities. No evidence of maternal toxicity was observed, but an increased abortion rate was observed in females that received 0.015 mg/kg/day rHuIFN-γ. No evidence of teratogenicity was observed in the fetuses available for examination.

3. Reproductive Study with rMuIFN-γ in the Mouse

Developmental toxicity of rMuIFN-γ was evaluated in pregnant mice treated with daily intramuscular injections of 0.15, 0.77, or 3.85 mg/kg (equivalent to 8×10^5, 4×10^6, and 2×10^7 U/kg) on days 6–15 of gestation (Kato *et al.,* 1990). Dams were either sacrificed on day 18 of gestation for standard teratological evaluation, or allowed to deliver offspring for subsequent postnatal evaluation. Maternal toxicity similar to that observed in the 28-day toxicity study was observed at the two higher doses. Abortions occurred in the high-dose females, and these dams either died or were killed in extremis on days 10–15; therefore, no fetal data were available for this group. Decreased postnatal viability was observed in the mid-dose group.

III. DISCUSSION

Recombinant human IFN-γ was one of the first highly species-specific recombinant proteins to be thoroughly assessed in the conventional safety models for xenobiotics. A complete series of acute and subchronic toxicity studies and segment I and II reproductive studies in the rat revealed no evidence of toxicity at any of the doses tested. Additionally, antibodies against the rHuIFN-γ were detected in the subchronic studies. The adverse effects observed in the clinic with cytokines are often exaggerated pharmacological effects of the molecules. Because the rat is pharmacologically nonresponsive to the activity of rHuIFN-γ, these results led many to conclude that the conventional test systems were inappropriate to evaluate the potential adverse effects of these types of molecules. Whereas these systems may be adequate to test the nonspecific toxic effects of the clinical formulations, they are not predictive of the toxicity related to the activity of the molecule. Because human interferons seem to have better activity in higher animal species (Adolf, 1985), several primate species were evaluated for toxicity. No toxicity was observed in acute or subchronic studies in marmosets or squirrel monkeys. Rhesus monkeys have been shown to be insensitive to the toxic effects of human interferons (Schellekens, 1982), and initial studies in cynomolgus monkeys also failed to demonstrate any adverse effects on body temperature or cardiovascular parameters. In contrast, chimpanzees exhibited a dose-related increase in body temperature with HuIFN-γ (Dawson *et al.,* 1983). Hematologic and hepatic toxicity has also been induced by HuIFN-γ in the chimpanzee (Schellekens *et al.,* 1984). These observations, together with preclinical experience with other interferons, has led some investigators to suggest that the chimpanzee is the best predictor of adverse effects in humans, and that other primate species are unreliable model systems (Fent and Zbinden, 1987). This conclusion is not supported, however, in the studies reviewed herein.

The toxicity profile for IFN-γ in humans is similar to that for IFN-α and IFN-β (Fent and Zbinden, 1987). The principal acute toxicity of the IFNs in humans consists of a flulike syndrome characterized by fever, chills, myalgias, arthralgias, and headaches (Scott *et al.,* 1981; Sherwin *et al.,* 1984; Quesada *et al.,* 1986; Mattson *et al.,* 1987). Fatigue is the most common chronic symptom. Hematologic toxicity consists mainly of leukopenia, but anemia and thrombocytopenia occur in some patients (Quesada *et al.,* 1986). Liver toxicity with elevation of serum transaminases and less frequently ALP or LDH is observed in some patients. Gastrointestinal toxicity is characterized by anorexia, nausea, vomiting, and diarrhea. Multidose studies in cynomolgus monkeys with rHuIFN-γ resulted in generalized systemic toxicity characterized by fever, lethargy, anorexia, and changes in hematology and serum chemistry values (Table XI), which are comparable to the changes observed in humans with interferon therapy. Mortality was observed at the highest dose in the monkey study. These data indicate that the cynomolgus monkey is responsive to the biological activities of human IFN-γ, and, if doses are escalated high enough, the potential clinical toxicity of the recombinant molecule can be characterized in this heterologous species. Histopathological lesions were induced in multiple organ systems and were consistent with known activities of IFN-γ. Hematotoxicity was characterized by depression of erythroid and myeloid elements in the peripheral blood and bone marrow, activities of IFN-γ that have been demonstrated both *in vitro* and *in vivo* (Mamus *et al.,* 1985; Naldini and Fleischmann, 1987). Lymphoid atrophy may be the result of the antiproliferative effect of IFN-γ on T and B lymphocytes (Keski-Oja and Moses, 1987). The pathogenic mechanism of lesion formation in the mucosa of the gastrointestinal tract is not as clearly evident, but it may also reflect a manifestation of the regulation of cell proliferation and differentiation exhibited by IFN-γ (Clemens and McNurlan, 1985). Hypertrophy and hyperplasia of the cells of the RES were evident in liver and spleen. Interferon-γ is a macrophage-activating factor, and the RE cell hyperplasia is consistent with a direct effect of rHuIFN-γ. Monkeys treated intramuscularly with rHuIFN-γ for the 90 days developed glomerulonephritis, which was morphologically compatible with an immune complex pathogenesis. These animals had detectable antibody titers against rHuIFN-γ, and it is possible that the glomerulonephritis was secondary to the antibody response against rHuIFN-γ. Antibodies to the rHuIFN-γ were generated in several of the species tested. This is not a problem in the homologous species (i.e., humans), and antibodies to rHuIFN-γ have not been detected in clinical studies (Fent and Zbin-

Table XI. Preclinical versus Clinical Experience with Interferon-γ[a]

Response	Cynomolgus monkey (rHuIFN-γ)	Mouse (rMuIFN-γ)	Human (rHuIFN-γ)
Constitutional symptoms			
Fever, anorexia, inactivity	+	±	+
Hematology/serum chemistry			
Neutropenia	+	−	+
Thrombocytopenia	+	−	+
Increased liver enzymes	+	+	+
Increased triglycerides	+	−	+
Decreased erythroid parameters	+	+	±
Increased LDH	+	+	+
Positive antibody response	+	−	−
Gross pathology			
Splenic enlargement	+	+	−
Testicular atrophy	−	+	−
Histopathology			
Activation of RES	+	+	NR[b]
Lymphoid depletion	+	±	NR
Bone marrow cellularity	+	+	NR
Hypospermatogenesis	+	+	NR
Liver atrophy/degeneration	+	±	NR
Glomerulonephritis	+	−	NR
GI tract lesions	+	+	NR
Exocrine/endocrine atrophy	−	+	NR
Cardiomyopathy	+	+	NR
Developmental/reproductive			
Abortifacient	+	+	NR
Altered estrus cyclicity	+	NR	NR

[a] A reference list is given in the text (see, in particular, Scott *et al.*, 1981; Sherwin *et al.*, 1984; Quesada *et al.*, 1986; Mattson *et al.*, 1987).

[b] NR, Not reported.

den, 1987; Kurzrock *et al.,* 1985). The neutralizing antibody response to rHuIFN-γ in the cynomolgus monkeys may have resulted in an amelioration of many of the effects of the treatment, because animals treated for 90 days did not exhibit the full spectrum of changes observed in those in the 4-week study.

Because rHuIFN-γ is not pharmacologically active in the mouse, a homologous recombinant murine IFN-γ was used in a subchronic toxicity study of 4 weeks duration. The result was a very close repetition of the pattern of toxicity observed in the cynomolgus monkey with rHuIFN-γ. The principal clinical chemistry and hematology changes were observed, except that no effect on neutrophils or platelets was seen in the mice. Histopathological changes were characterized by diffuse hyperplasia of the RES, lymphoid atrophy, and testicular atrophy. Other lesions observed in both the mouse and monkey included changes in bone marrow cellularity, gastrointestinal tract lesions, and cardiomyopathy. Additional lesions in the mice that were not present in monkeys were observed in several endocrine and exocrine glands and were characterized by atrophic changes. Glomerulonephritis was not observed in mice treated with rMuIFN-γ, however, the mice did not develop antibodies to the rMuIFN-γ.

Reproductive studies in monkeys with rHuIFN-γ and in mice with rMuIFN-γ indicated that both molecules are potential abortifacients. No evidence of this activity was observed in rats treated with rHuIFN-γ. The lack of reproductive toxicity of rHuIFN-γ in rats is not surprising in view of the known lack of biological activity of the human molecule in this species. This activity appears to represent a direct pharmacological activity of the IFN-γ in responsive species.

IV. SUMMARY

Interferon-γ is a highly species-specific cytokine and has the most restricted host range of activity of the interferons. Recombinant human IFN-γ was one of the first species-specific recombinant proteins to be thoroughly assessed in conventional safety models used for xenobiotics. Acute single-dose intravenous toxicity studies with rHuIFN-γ were performed in rats, marmosets, and squirrel monkeys with no indications of toxicity. A complete series of subchronic toxicity studies and segment I and II reproductive studies in the rat revealed no evidence of toxicity at any of the doses tested. These results suggested that studies conducted in pharmacologically nonresponsive species may not be predictive of clinical toxicity. Human IFN-γ is active on nonhuman primate cells, though not at the same level as on human cells. Multidose studies in cynomolgus monkeys with rHuIFN-γ for 28 or 90 days were predictive of many of the dose-limiting clinical toxicities. Qualitative similarity was observed between toxicity studies employing rHuIFN-γ in the cynomolgus monkey and rMuIFN-γ in the mouse. The adverse effects seen in toxicity studies with cytokines and growth factors are often exaggerated pharmacological effects of the molecules, and therefore can only be studied in a responsive species. In situations in which a high degree of species specificity is encountered, studies employing a recombinant protein in a homologous species may provide a useful test system for preclinical safety assessment.

Acknowledgments

The material reviewed includes experimental studies conducted at several facilities to support registration of Actimmune (recombinant human interferon-γ). For the provision of histological sections for photomicrographs we wish to thank Dr. Tadao Suzuki of Daiichi Pharmaceutical Co., Ltd. For their contributions to this research program we thank Dr. M. Kikumori and Dr. M. Nomora of Daiichi, and Dr. M. Saitoh and Dr. M. Nagatani of Hamamatsu Seigiken Research, and Dr. D. Goeddel, Dr. S. Kramer, Dr. H. Jaffe, Dr. P. Working, and M. Lewandowski of Genentech, Inc.

References

Adolf, G. R. (1985). *Oncology* **42**, Suppl. 1, 33–40.

Branca, B. A., and Baglioni, C. (1981). *Nature (London)* **294**, 768–770.

Clemens, M. J., and McNurlan, M. A. (1985). *Biochem. J.* **226**, 345–360.

Dawson, A. F., Gerlis, L., Otto, B., de Reus, A., and Schellekens, H. (1983). *In* "Interferons" (T. Kishida, ed.), pp. 357–361. ISFN, Kyoto.

Dijkema, R., van der Meide, P. H., Pouwels, P. H., Caspers, M., Dubbeld, M., and Schellekens, H. (1985). *EMBO J.* **4**, 761–767.

Farrar, W. L., Johnson, H. M., and Farrar, J. J. (1981). *J. Immunol.* **126**, 1120–1125.

Fent, K., and Zbinden, G. (1987). *Trends Pharmacol. Sci.* **8**, 100–105.

Ghezzi, P., and Dinarello, C. A. (1988). *J. Immunol.* **140**, 4238–4244.

Goeddel, D. V., Leung, D. W., Dull, T. J., Gross, M., Lawn, R. M., McCandliss, R., Seeburg, P. H., Ullich, A., Yelverton, E., and Gray, P. W. (1981). *Nature (London)* **290**, 20–26.

Gray, P. W., and Goeddel, D. V. (1982). *Nature (London)* **298**, 859–863.

Gray, P. W., and Goeddel, D. V. (1983). *Proc. Natl. Acad. Sci. U.S.A.* **80**, 5842–5846.

Gray, P. W., Leung, D. W., Pennica, D., Yelverton, E., Najarian, R., Simonsen, C. C., Derynck, R., Sherwook, P. J., Wallace, D. M., Berger, S. L., Levinson, A. D., and Goeddel, D. V. (1982). *Nature (London)* **295**, 503–508.

Haq, A. U., Rinehart, J. J., and Maca, R. D. (1985). *J. Leukocyte Biol.* **38**, 735–746.

Hayes, T. J. (1990). *In* "Preclinical Evaluation of Peptides and Recombinant Proteins" (A. Sundwall, L. Ekman, H.-E. Johansson, B. Sjöberg, and I. Sjöholm, eds.), pp. 15–18. Assoc. Swed. Pharm. Ind. Stockholm.

Kato, I., Kimura, S., Furuhashi, T., Nakayoshi, H., Takayama, S., and Uenishi, N. (1990). *Fundam. Appl. Toxicol.* **14**, 658–665.

Keski-Oja, J., and Moses, H. L. (1987). *Med. Biol.* **65**, 13–20.

Kurzrock, R., Rosenblum, M. G., Sherwin, S. A., Rios, A., Talpaz, M., Quesada, J. R., and Gutterman, J. U. (1985). *Oncology* **42**, Suppl. 1, 41–50.

Lewandowski, M. E., Working, P. K., Osterburg, I., Vogel, F., Korte, R., and Green, J. D. (1991). *Toxicologist* **11**, 343.

Mamus, S. W., Beck-Schroeder, S., and Zanjani, E. D. (1985). *J. Clin. Invest.* **75**, 1496–1503.

Mattson, K., Holsti, L. R., Niiranen, A., Pyrhönen, S., Färkkilä, M., Härtel, G., Standertskiöld-Nordenstam, C.-G., and Cantell, K. (1987). *In* "The Biology of the Interferon System 1986" (K. Cantell and H. Schellekens, eds.), pp. 387–397. Nijhoff, Boston.

Naldini, A., and Fleischmann, W. R., Jr. (1987). *J. Biol. Response Modif.* **6**, 546–555.

Naylor, S. L., Sakaguchi, A. Y., Shows, T. B., Law, M. L., Goeddel, D. V., and Gray, P. W. (1983). *J. Exp. Med.* **157**, 1020–1027.

Owerbach, D., Rutter, W. J., Shows, T. B., Gray, P., Goeddel, D. V., and Lawn, R. M. (1981). *Proc. Natl. Acad. Sci. U.S.A.* **78**, 3123–3127.

Quesada, J. R., Talpaz, M., Rios, A., Kurzrock, R., and Gutterman, J. U. (1986). *J. Clin. Oncol.* **4**, 234–243.

Remick, D. G., and Kunkel, S. L. (1989). *Lab. Invest.* **60**, 317–319.

Schellekens, H. (1982). *In* "Interferons" (T. C. Memgan and R. M. Friedman, eds.), Vol. 25, pp. 387–392.

Schellekens, H., de Reus, A., and Meide, P. H. (1984). *J. Med. Primatol.* **13**, 235–245.

Schreiber, R. D., and Celada, A. (1985). *In* "Lymphokines" (E. Pick and M. Landy, eds.), Vol. 11, pp. 87–118. Academic Press, New York.

Scott, G. M., Secher, D. S., Flowers, D., Bate, J., Cantell, K., and Tyrrell, D. A. J. (1981). *Br. Med. J. No. 282,* 1345–1348.

Sherwin, S. A., Foon, K. A., Abrams, P. G., Heyman, M. R., Ochs, J. J., Watson, T., Maluish, A., and Oldham, R. K. (1984). *J. Biol. Response Modif.* **3,** 599–607.

Stewart, W. E. (1979). "The Interferon System," pp. 13–45. Springer Publ., New York.

Teelmann, K., Hohbach, C., and Lehmann, H. (1986). *Arch. Toxicol.* **59,** 195–200.

Trown, P. W., Wills, R. J., and Kamm, J. J. (1986). *Cancer (Philadelphia)* **57,** 1648–1656.

Vilcek, J., Kelker, H. C., Le, J., and Yip, Y. K. (1985). *In* "Mediators in Cell Growth and Differentiation" (R. J. Ford and A. L. Maizel, eds.), Vol. 37, pp. 299–313. Raven, New York.

Wheelock, E. F. (1965). *Science* **149,** 310–311.

Section II
CYTOKINE RECEPTORS

Introduction to Cytokine Receptors: Structure and Signal Transduction

Brian Foxwell and Kathy Barrett
Sunley Research Institute
London, England

I. INTRODUCTION

Common features of all cytokines are the low concentration needed to elicit their effects and the diverse range of biologic activities. It has been evident for some time that cytokines transmit their biological signals to responsive cells by interaction with specific high-affinity cell surface receptors. Investigations were difficult because of the low expression of cytokine receptors, which are rarely expressed above a few hundred per cell. However, during the last 5 years very rapid progress has been made in the biological characterization of these receptors.

The availability of recombinant cytokines coincided with the development of advanced cloning technologies. One of the first cytokine receptors purified was the IL-2R α chain (TAC) using standard immunoaffinity protein purification technology, followed by protein sequencing, generation of oligonucleotide probes, and screening of cDNA libraries. Similar techniques have been used for the cloning of human tumor necrosis factor (TNF) R and human interferon-γ (IFN-γ) R. However, the majority of the cytokine receptors have been cloned using expression cloning techniques where a mammalian cell line, transfected with a cDNA library, has been screened either by antibodies to the receptor, e.g., IL-2R β chain; by biotinylated cytokine, e.g., for IL-6 receptor; by radiolabeled cytokine, for IL-7, IL-3, IL-5, receptors; or by subtraction library, e.g., IL-4R. Often, the cloning of either the human or murine receptor has led to the isolation of its counterpart using lower stringency screening with cDNA probes derived from the cloned version of the receptor.

The cloning of many receptors has led to the observation that the majority of the receptors fall into one of three families: (1) the tumor necrosis factor receptors (TNFR); (2) the hematopoietic growth factor receptor family (HGFRF); (3) the immunoglobulin (Ig) supergene family.

International Review of Experimental Pathology, Volume 34B

Some receptors, e.g., IL-2R α chain and IFN-γ receptor, do not belong to any grouping. Within each family, most cytokine receptors show functional as well as structural common traits. The HGFRF are proteins responsible for the binding of a single cytokine, although many receptors require an additional protein to confer high affinity [IL-2R, IL-3R, IL-5R, granulocyte-macrophage colony stimulating factor (GM-CSFR), and IL-6R]. The two most well-characterized receptors of the TNF group show multiple binding chains and multiple ligands (TNFRs and nerve growth factor receptor (NGFR)/tropomyosin receptor kinase (trk). The IL-1R, a member of the Ig supergene family, comprises two receptors and three ligands (IL-1a, IL-1b, and IL-1 receptor antagonist).

There is little knowledge of the mechanisms by which cytokines transmit signals via their receptors. Cloning of the receptor cDNAs revealed that there is usually no obvious enzymatic mechanism within the receptor structure and thus auxiliary molecules are thought to play a role, e.g., gp130 which is associated with the IL-6R. However, even the gp130 does not have any known intrinsic enzyme activity. There seems to be no obvious common signal transduction mechanism within a given family.

For the purposes of this review, we have dealt with the receptor groups by highlighting the individual members in each case. The review is confined to receptor structure and signaling.

II. TUMOR NECROSIS FACTOR RECEPTOR FAMILY

This group of cytokine receptors comprises proteins with structural similarities to the two TNF receptors. The family is at present smaller than the HGFRF, and only the TNF receptors would normally be regarded as cytokine receptors. In addition to the two TNFRs, the family includes the low-affinity nerve growth factor receptor (L-NGFR) (81), the B cell antigen CD40 (145), and several proteins likely to be receptors, but which have no defined ligands: the T cell antigens OX40 (98) and CD27 (18); the Fas antigen expressed on myeloid; T lymphoblastoid and fibroblast cells (78); and CD30, a marker for tumor cell lines derived from patients with Hodgkin's lymphoma (32). Two other members, an open reading frame from Shope fibroma virus (SFV-T2) (161) and 4-1BB, a cDNA clone isolated from human T cells (91), have not been identified as proteins *in vivo*.

The structural definition of this family lies with an arrangement of three or four conserved cysteine rich sequences of approximately 40 amino acids in the extracellular domains. In some of the family members, one or more of the repeats are truncated as in the p55 TNFR and the Fas antigen. In the main, there is no homology in the cytoplasmic domains of these proteins except for a region of 44 amino acids with sequence similarity present in the intracellular domains of Fas antigen, p55 TNFR, and CD40 (78). This region spans sequences that appear to be essential for receptor signaling in CD40 (74) and the p55 TNFR (16). Apart from this observation, no identifiable regions for signaling functions, e.g., kinases, have been described in any of these proteins. From the studies made on the two family members for which ligands exist, TNFRs and L-NGFR, it would appear that their receptors form complex systems, binding more than one ligand and exhibiting multiple receptors for a given ligand.

A. TNF Receptors

From earlier studies there were indications that the TNF system was complex. Both TNF (TNF-α) and a second cytokine, lymphotoxin (LT/TNFβ) exhibited very similar activities, i.e., proinflammation, cytotoxicity, and induction of CD25 (13). The main difference between the two cytokines is their source, TNF being mainly myeloid in origin (52,123,144,157), whereas LT is mainly T cell derived (26,107,115,147). Receptor binding studies on these cytokines led to the observation that they cross-competed each other (1), and affinity cross-linking identified binding moieties of 55 and 75 kDa expressed on the cell surface (143,146). Binding studies on both receptors identified a single affinity receptor with K_d of 10^{-10}–$10^{-11} M$ (70). Cloning of their receptors led to the isolation of two proteins normally termed p55 (or p60) TNFR (57,95,129) and p75 (or p80) TNFR (137). Both receptors are able to bind TNF and LT, and cellular expression of the transfected receptor cDNA displays dual affinity binding. The observation that TNF has two distinct receptors led to speculation that they may be responsible for the pleiotropy (multiple effects) of TNF and LT. Preliminary evidence from studies on murine cell lines where only one or other of the receptors is expressed (11,151) or transfection studies using the human p55 R (16,150) suggests that this might be the case, with the p55 TNFR mediating cytotoxic function and the p75 receptor mediating growth-promoting activity. However, studies on the expression of both receptors in various tissues have indicated that the two forms are normally coexpressed (17,70). Both TNFRs also exist in soluble forms which have been identified *in vivo* (36,110,131). The formation of sTNFR appears to be by proteolytic cleavage of the mature cell surface receptor (116) in a manner akin to the generation of sIL-2R α chain (124).

The nature of the TNFR signaling is quite different from what has so far been observed with the HGFRF. First, both TNF and LT exist as trimers and would appear to bind receptors as such (34,82,142). Second, unlike the HGFRF, anti-receptor antibodies can be agonistic as well as antagonistic (35,37). This has led to speculation that receptor aggregation is a requirement for signaling, a hypothesis supported by the observation that antagonistic antibodies lose their stimulatory properties when used as Fab monomers (35). The involvement of G proteins has been suggested from the induction of GTP binding activity and the inhibiting effects of pertussis toxin on TNF effects (73). This is followed by the elevation of cAMP (170) and, indeed, pharmacological agents which increase intracellular cAMP concentrations have rendered cells more sensitive to TNF toxicity (20). TNF also activates a serine kinase, causing the phosphorylation of serine residues of the p26/p28 heat shock proteins (7,130). The involvement of tyrosine kinases in TNFR signaling, however, is unclear, with contrary evidence being reported (29,90). Several mechanisms by which TNF induces cytotoxicity have been proposed (reviewed in 92), including reports that direct microinjection of TNF can elicit a response (141), thus indicating that receptors are not always required for cytotoxic activity. However, this could not be reproduced in all TNF responsive cell types and would be at odds with the existence of agonistic anti-receptor antibodies.

B. Low Affinity Nerve Growth Factor Receptor

NGF initiates the differentiation and survival of selective neuronal populations. The biological activity of NGF is mediated by a high-affinity receptor $(K_d \sim 10^{-11}M)$ expressed on responsive cell lines, while nonresponsive lines exhibit only a low-affinity receptor $(K_d \sim 10^{-9}M)$ (59). Cloning of the NGFR revealed a 75-kDa molecule, which exhibited low-affinity binding (L-NGFR) (81). Cross-linking studies revealed that a second protein was involved in the high-affinity receptor, and this was identified as the proto-onocogene tropomyosin receptor kinase (64,88), a tyrosine kinase which alone may also bind NGF with high affinity (88). The NGFR also binds other ligands: brain derived neurotrophic factor (BDNF), neurotrophin-3 (NT-3), and NT-4. The specificity of binding of these ligands is determined by the association of LNGFR with different members of the trk family (24,89). The association of tyrosine kinase activity with the LNGFR provides an obvious mechanism of signal transduction, and NGF activation of tyrosine phosphorylation has been observed (12,84). Receptor aggregation also appears to be important in signaling function, since NGF responsive cells have their receptors preaggregated, whereas they are dispersed on nonresponsive cells (164). NGF also activates protein kinase C, causing the inhibition of a second kinase, Nsp 100 kinase (60).

C. Other TNFR Family Members

Agonistic antibodies stimulate other TNFR family members, which suggests that receptor self association is required for signaling. CD40 appears to be linked to tyrosine kinase activity during B cell ontogeny (159). The CD40 ligand was recently defined as a T cell surface antigen capable of inducing the proliferation of splenic or tonsillar B cells and the secretion of IgE by IL-4-stimulated B cells (6), while antibodies to CD40 also function with IL-4 in driving the release of soluble CD23 (22) and in reversing the inhibitory effects of anti-CD19 antibodies, TGF-β, and IFN-γ on IL-4 activity (54). The full characterization of the other family members must await the identification of their active ligands. It is interesting to note that the recombinantly expressed SFV-T2 protein can bind TNF (138).

III. THE HEMATOPOIETIC GROWTH FACTOR RECEPTOR FAMILY

The hematopoietic growth factor receptor family contains the majority of cytokine receptors. This family contains receptors for IL-2 (β chain), IL-3, IL-4, IL-5, IL-7, GM-CSF, and leukocyte inhibition factor (LIF). The IL-6R and G-CSFR also have characteristics of the HGFRF as well as the Ig gene superfamily and thus will also be considered in this section. The HGFRF also includes proteins that do not bind ligand but form part of the receptor structure, i.e., the gp130 (IL-6R β chain) and the common β chain of the IL-3, IL-5, and GM-CSF receptors.

The basic characteristics of this family are conserved cysteine residues in the extracellular domain and a pentameric tryptophan–serine–X–tryptophan–serine motif—where X is any amino acid—just proximal to the transmembrane domain. The significance of this motif is unknown, but deletion of both trp residues from the IL-2R β chain renders the receptor inactive. The receptors do show a varying degree of homology in their extracellular domains, but very little in the cytosolic domains. The cytosolic domains contain no identifiable kinase or other enzymatic function. It is possible that other receptor-associated proteins perform this task (see below). Functionally, these receptors each bind only one ligand, and the majority display both high- and low-affinity receptors, although the structural reason for the dual affinities varies between different receptors.

A. IL-2 Receptor

IL-2, the major T cell growth factor, was one of the first cytokines characterized (reviewed in 139,140,165). The receptors for IL-2 display many HGFRF characteristics with both high affinity ($K_d \sim 10^{-11}\ M$) and low affinity ($K_d \sim 10^{-8} M$) receptors being expressed (120). The basis of dual affinity lies in the heterodimeric structure of the receptor. The high-affinity receptor comprises the IL-2R β chain (p70) (14,31,63,121,126,134,153,166) in conjunction with the smaller p55 α chain (CD25), characterized much earlier and originally known as the TAC protein (25,94,100). The α chain is not part of the HGFRF and has a short six amino acid cytoplasmic tail and appears to be unable to transmit any intracellular signal. On activated T cells, it is normally expressed at a 10-fold excess over the β chain and on its own comprises the low-affinity receptor (97,120,121). The biological significance of these receptors is unknown, but proteolytic cleavage of the IL-2R α chain gives rise to soluble receptors (sIL-2R) (124). Alone, the β chain also binds IL-2, with an intermediate affinity of $K_d \sim 10^{-9} M$ (63,97,121,156). The high affinity of the heterodimer is obtained by combination of the fast association kinetics of the α chain coupled with the low dissociation kinetics of the β chain (97). Both the $\alpha\beta$ chain dimer and the β chain alone are internalized on the binding ligand and can mediate IL-2 activity (63,119,135,156,168). However, the failure of the cloned β chain to bind IL-2 when expressed in isolation in fibroblast cells (155) has given rise to speculation on the existence of a third, γ chain of the IL-2R. Several reports have claimed to have identified such a protein (66,126,127,133,155).

The key role of the IL-2/IL-2R in T and B cell proliferation has led to considerable study of its signaling mechanism. The IL-2R does not utilize the dual second messenger pathway of inositol triphosphate (IP3)/Ca^{2+} and diacylglycerol/protein kinase C (101,154,163), originating from the cleavage of phosphatidyl inositol bis-phosphate, used by the T cell receptor. It has been reported that IL-2 can induce the generation of a myristiated diacylglycerol and inositol phosphate glycan from the hydrolysis of inositol glycolipid (33). The involvement of tyrosine kinase activation has been reported by several groups (41,77,99,125), and IL-2 induces tyrosine phosphorylation of the IL-2R β chain (8,132) and the serine phosphorylation of CD45 (162). Moreover, the tyrosine kinase proto-oncogene p56lck has been found in association with the IL-2R β chain (62). IL-2 has also been shown to be able to activate p21ras (56,80,128) and G proteins (39), the c-raf serine/threonine kinase (171), and IP3 kinase (10,117). In the nucleus, IL-2 has been shown to induce c-myb (21), c-fos, and c-myc (23). However, the extent of the involvement of any of these observed intracellular biochemical changes to the IL-2R signal transduction pathway and their relationship to one another has yet to be established.

B. The IL-4 and IL-7 Receptors

These cytokines are growth factors for activated T cells, but were originally described as B cell growth factors acting on mature (IL-4) and immature (IL-7) cells (27,65). Like all cytokines, they display a great deal of pleiotropy; for example, IL-4 induces CD23 and surface IgM expression (118) on B cells and IL-6 production on endothelial cells (71), but blocks LPS-induced TNF and IL-1 production by monocytes (38,167), whereas IL-7 can induce the production of these inflammatory cytokines by monocytes (4) and also induce CD25 expression of T cells (65).

The IL-4 receptor has been identified and cloned as $\sim$140-kDa molecule displaying a single high-affinity binding ($K_d \sim 10^{-10}M$) (48,61,72,103). A low-affinity receptor ($K_d \sim 3 \times 10^{-8}M$) has been identified on human peripheral blood mononuclear cells (44) where cross-linking studies suggested that the low-affinity binding was due to the presence of a putative 65/75-kDa protein associated with the IL-4R. A low-affinity IL-4 binding activity has also been isolated from culture supernatants (5). However, these lower molecular weight IL-4R-associated proteins may be, in part, proteolytic products of the main receptor protein (85). The existence of high-affinity sIL-4R has been identified in murine tissue fluids (40), which is probably the product of an alternative splicing of IL-4R mRNA to produce a soluble truncated receptor (103). However, the existence of such a sIL-4R mRNA has not been identified in human cells (72).

The IL-7R also expresses a dual affinity with a high ($K_d \sim 5 \times 10^{-11}M$) and a low ($K_d \sim 10^{-9}M$) binding (53,114). Park et $al.$ (114) have suggested that the dual affinity is due to negative cooperativity of IL-7 binding, and thus is observed when the cloned human or murine IL-7R is expressed in COS fibroblast cells (53). A low affinity ($K_d > 10^{-8}M$) IL-7R is also expressed on COS fibroblast cells but this appears to be the function of some other as yet uncharacterized receptor (53). The cloned fibroblast derived IL-7R cannot be affinity cross-linked to IL-7 (53). However, the technique easily detects the IL-7R on human T cells (45). On human T cells, the IL-7R undergoes changes following T cell activation, being downregulated, and with a smaller "second" form of receptor appearing. The expression of the novel receptor is found on all T cells that can respond to IL-7 as a growth factor (45). Whether this second IL-7R is due to an alternative receptor or is the product of a different splicing of mRNA from a single gene is unclear. Alternatively spliced products of the cloned human IL-7R have been identified (53), producing a putative sIL-7R and a smaller membrane-bound form.

Receptor signaling studies on these molecules have shown little in common with each other or the IL-2R. IL-4-induced upregulation of CD23 in human tonsillar B cells appears to require Ca^{2+} IP3 and cAMP signals (42,118). However, such mechanisms have not been identified in murine B cells or human B cell lines displaying the same IL-4 function (42,49). These signals, however, are not used by IL-4 to induce sIgM (118). This, with other evidence, has led to speculation that the upregulation of CD23 and sIgM in human B cells is operated by different IL-4Rs and/or signal pathways. Unlike IL-2, IL-4 does not induce p21ras activity (128), and the utilization of tyrosine kinase by this receptor is disputed in the published literature (9,75). However, the existence of multiple signaling mechanisms may account for these discrepancies.

The utilization of tyrosine kinases by IL-4R has been reported in mature T cells, lymphoblastic leukemia T cells, thymocytes, and B cells

(28,122,158,160). The generation of IP3 by IL-7 has been reported (28,158,160) in the latter three cells types, but a more recent study in thymocytes and mature T cells has not confirmed this (122). No increases in intracellular Ca^{2+} associated with the function of IP3 have been reported (122).

C. IL-3, IL-5, and GM-CSF Receptors

These receptors share a common β chain. IL-3 or GM-CSF are potent hematopoietic growth factors stimulating the proliferation and differentiation of various lineages of hematopoietic cells, including multipotent stem cells and lineage cells. In the human system, IL-5 has also been reported to effect basophils; however, the effects of IL-5 on B cell function are thus far confined to the murine system. These cytokines can all influence eosinophilopoiesis, with IL-5 being the most potent. Binding and cross-linking studies had indicated that IL-3 and GM-CSF could partially cross-compete each other's binding and suggested the presence of common structural elements for both receptors (113). These receptors and IL-5R all display dual affinity with high-affinity receptors of $K_d \sim 10^{-10}\ M$ and low-affinity receptors of $K_d 10^{-8}-10^{-7}\ M$ (51,113,149). The recent cloning of the proteins comprising the high- and low-affinity receptors for these cytokines has revealed the existence of heterodimeric receptor structures. In the human system, the smaller α chains ($\sim$70 kDa) of IL-3 (87) GM-CSF (51), and IL-5 (152) receptors alone express low-affinity binding and are specific for each cytokine. The high affinity is the result of association of each α chain with a common β chain (140 kDa) shared by all three receptors, which alone does not bind the cytokines (87,152). As a refinement of this system, a second β chain, AIC 2A, has been identified as a component of the murine IL-3R (79); this protein shares 95% sequence homology with the common β chain, AIC 2B (55,86,87), of the murine IL-3, IL-5, (149), and GM-CSF receptors. Unlike AIC2B, the AIC2A molecule binds IL-3 with low affinity (79). The comparative utilization of AIC 2A and AIC 2B by the high-affinity murine IL-3R is unclear.

Studies on the receptor signaling mechanism have shown that IL-3, IL-5, and GM-CSF induce the tyrosine phosphorylation of a similar set of cytoplasmic proteins (9,105). Studies have also indicated that the β chain of the IL-3R can be phosphorylated on tyrosine (76). IL-3 and GM-CSF, like IL-2, are also capable of inducing the activation of p21ras (128).

D. The IL-6 Receptor

As with other cytokines, cloning and expression of purified IL-6 has led to identification of many functions, including growth and differentiation activities on B cells, myeloma-plasmacytomas, T cells, hepatocytes, and hematopoietic stem cells. The IL-6R shows dual affinity binding with high-affinity receptors of $K_d \sim 10^{-11} M$ and low-affinity receptors of $K_d \sim 10^{-9} M$ (169). The cloning of an 80-kDa receptor protein revealed structural elements of both the HGFRF and the Ig supergene family (169). Further studies on the IL-6R structure revealed the existence of an auxiliary signaling molecule: gp130 (IL-6R β chain) (148). This protein associates with the IL-6R/IL-6 complex and converts the receptor from low-affinity to high-affinity binding (67). Cloning of the gp130 molecule has also identified this protein as a member of the HGFRF (67). The involvement of the gp130 protein in IL-6R signaling was demonstrated by the observation that genetically engineered sIL-6R was capable, when complexed with IL-6, of association with gp130 and the subsequent manifestation of IL-6 activity (148). Since sIL-6R is also produced naturally (108), there is the possible prospect that cells, only expressing the gp130 but not IL-6R, could be affected by sIL-6R/IL-6 complexes. Recently, it has been reported that gp130 could also serve, like the β chain of the IL-3, IL-5, and GM-CSF receptors, as an auxiliary protein for the oncostatin M and LIF receptors (50). Regardless of its signaling role, the gp130 does not encode any kinase or known signaling function, although it does possess a GTP binding motif, but this can be deleted without affecting function (104). In fact, little is known of how the IL-6 transduces its signals or what second messenger system might be employed. However, IL-6 induces the tyrosine phosphorylation of the gp130 (104).

E. G-CSF Receptor

Granulocyte colony stimulating factor, secreted by macrophages, fibroblasts, and endothelial cells, was originally identified by its ability to stimulate *in vitro* the survival, proliferation, and differentiation of predominantly neutrophilic granulocytes from bone marrow progenitors. This factor has now been shown to affect mature neutrophils, inducing alkaline phosphatase, high-affinity IgA Fc receptors, priming for respiratory burst, and increased chemotaxis. G-CSF has also been reported to have proliferative effects on some myeloid leukemic cells and adenocarcinomas and small lung carcinomas. Cloning of the receptor for this cytokine identified, in the human, two integral membrane proteins of 759 and 812 amino acids produced from a single gene by the alternatively spliced mRNAs, the two products differing in the length of their cytoplasmic domains (93,106). The mouse appears to produce only the larger version of the receptor (47). Like the IL-6R, the G-CSFR has structural relationship with the HGFRF and the Ig superfamily, and, in addition, with fibronectin type III (93). The cytoplasmic domains of murine G-CSF and IL-4 receptor show a reasonable degree of homology (47). Both the cloned and native receptor, like other HGFRF members, show dual high affinity ($K_d \sim 2$–$5 \times 10^{-10} M$) and low affinity ($2 \times 10^{-9} M$) (46).

F. Other Family Members

As stated, the HGFRF includes receptors such as those for prolactin and erythropoietin (EPO) that are not classically considered to be cytokines and as such will not be dealt with here in any detail. The importance of many of these cytokines would suggest a latent potential for the HGFRF to act as oncogenes. In this respect, Longmore and co-workers (96) have recently shown that a mutant EPOR that has a point mutation in codon 129, converting arginine to cysteine, can transmit a growth signal in the absence of ligand, and injection of retrovirus encoding this receptor variant into mice produces erythrocytosis and splenomegaly.

IV. THE IMMUNOGLOBULIN SUPERGENE FAMILY

This group of receptors includes many tyrosine kinase-expressing receptors: e.g., receptors for platelet-derived growth factor (PDGF), epidermal growth factor (EGF), insulin and insulin-like growth factors (IGF); the receptor for colony stimulating factor-1 (c-fms); and the Steel factor receptor, c-kit. Several of these receptors have also been identified as proto-oncogenes, where mutated forms of the receptor have permanently activated tyrosine kinase activity. Some of these receptors, PDGF, EGF, and IGF, are heterogenous, with more than one form of receptor existing, e.g., PDGFRα and β, which can combine in different forms, aa, ab, or bb. In the case of the insulin receptor system, insulin, IGF-1, and IGF-2 can cross-bind each other's receptors to a certain degree. The function and structure of these receptors has been reviewed extensively elsewhere. However, the second subclass of this family includes what is best described as the IL-1/IL-1R system including three separate ligands and possibly up to three separate receptors. The IL-1Rs have no tyrosine kinase function in the cytoplasmic domain.

The IL-1 Receptor System

IL-1 consists of two separate ligands, IL-1a and IL-1b. They have a low amino acid identity (26%) but bind to the same cell surface receptors to induce a wide range of activities: stimulation of thymocyte proliferation, accessory factor for T cell activation; stimulation of hematopoietic cell growth and differentiation; and induction of acute phase protein synthesis and induction of prostaglandin and collagenase synthesis by fibroblasts and chondrocytes (111). Recently, a third ligand IRAP (IL-1 receptor agonist protein) has been identified which acts as a naturally occurring receptor antagonist, binding with an affinity similar to that of the agonistic ligands, but being unable on binding to transmit any biological signal (19). Characterization of the IL-1R has identified two separate moieties (15). The molecular cloning has resulted in the identification of an 80-kDa form of the receptor that is expressed on T cells and fibroblasts and displays a single class of high-affinity receptors ($K_d \sim 2 \times 10^{-10}\,M$) (136). However, a very high affinity form ($K_d \sim 5 \times 10^{-12}\,M$) has also been reported on murine T cells and human keratinocytes (30). A second receptor of small size (p60) has been identified on B cells; this receptor appears to display dual affinity binding with high ($K_d \sim 5 \times 10^{-11}\,M$) and low ($K_d \sim 10^{-9}\,M$) affinity receptors (15). Unlike the TNFR system, the IL-1R appears to be cell lineage specific and both forms of IL-1, a and b, bind both forms of the receptor with dual affinities. The third ligand, IRAP, also binds IL-1 p80 and p60 with an affinity the same as that of the agonistic ligands. Binding of this molecule does not induce IL-1R internalization or IL-1 induced EGFR phosphorylation.

Signaling by IL-1 has been extensively studied; however, there is no consensual agreement on what mechanism IL-1 uses to signal (102,109). Studies have reportedly shown that IL-1 signaling is linked to the activation of a G protein and the elevation of cAMP, thus triggering protein kinase A and culminating in activation of the NFkB transcription factor (102). However, others have been unable to reproduce the utilization of cAMP and PKA by IL-1R, although the activation of uncharacterized kinases has been reported with the induction of the serine phosphorylation of EGFR, IL-1R, and hsp27 (109). An interesting observation on the IL-1R is the ability to produce profound biological effects at very low (~1%) receptor occupancy (30). The IL-1/IL-1R complex has been found in the nucleus but whether this implies a direct affect of IL-1 on the regulation of target cell DNA is uncertain.

V. OTHER CYTOKINE RECEPTORS

IL-2R α Chain and IFN-γR

While the majority of cytokine receptors fall into one of the three families described, there are two notable exceptions, IL-2R α chain and IFN-γR. The IL-2R α chain was the first cytokine receptor to be identified and cloned, and its role and involvement in IL-2R structure and function have already been discussed (Section I). The receptor for IFN-γ also shows no homology to other receptors, or any other known protein. IFN-γ has antiviral activity and effects T cell differentiation, macrophage activity, and upregulation of class II MHC expression, and also inhibits the function of IL-4. The IFN-γR has been characterized and cloned from murine and human cells as a 90-kDa protein (2,3,58) and appears to bind IFN-γ as a dimer (43). In common with other cytokine receptors, it has no obvious means of transducing signals, and thus it is assumed that other proteins are associated with the ligand binding chain to form the active receptor. Recent studies have indicated that a species-specific accessory factor(s) is required for receptor signaling. In human, at least one of these factors appears to be encoded by chromosome 21q (68,83) and in mouse by a gene on chromosome 16 (69).

Signal transduction studies on the IFN-γR have implicated several second messenger systems, including G proteins and adenylate cyclase, cAMP, calcium ion flux and protein kinase C (112), protein phosphorylation, and Na$^+$/H$^+$ exchange (112) in the functioning of this receptor.

References

1. Aggarwal, B. B., Eessalu, T. E., and HAss, P. E. (1985). *Nature (London)* **318**, 665–667.
2. Aguet, M., Dembic, Z., and Merlin, G. (1988). *Cell* **55**(2), 273–280.
3. Aguet, M., and Merlin, G. (1987). *J. Exp. Med.* **165**(4), 988–999.
4. Alderson, M. R., Tough, T. W., Ziegler, S. F., and Grabstein, K. H. (1991). *J. Exp. Med.* **173**(4), 923–930.
5. Armitage, R. J., Clifford, K., Spriggs, M. K., MacDuff, B. M., Dower, S. K., Rauch, C. M., Van Ness, K., March, C. J., and Fanslow, W. C. (1991). *J. Cell. Biochem.* **15F** (Suppl.), 111.
6. Armitage, R. J., Fanslow, W. C., Strockbine, L., Sato, T. A., Clifford, K. N., Macduff, B. M., Anderson, D. M., Gimpel, S. D., Davis-Smith, T., Maliszewski, C. R., Clark, E. A., Smith, C. A., Grabstein, K. H., Cosman, D., and Spriggs, M. K. *Nature (London)* **357**, 80–82.
7. Arrigo, A. P. (1990). *Mol. Cell. Biol.* **10**(3), 1276–1280. [Published erratum appears in *Mol. Cell. Biol.* (1990). **10**(7), 3857].
8. Asao, H., Takeshita, T., Nakamura, M., Nagata, K., and Sugamura, K. (1990). *J. Exp. Med.* **171**(3), 637–644. [published erratum appears in *J. Exp. Med.* **(1990). 171**(6), 2183].
9. Augustine, J. A., Schlager, J. W., and Abraham, R. T. (1990). *Biochem. Biophys. Acta.* **1052**(2), 313–322.
10. Augustine, J. A., Sutor, S. L., and Abraham, R. T. (1991). *Mol. Cell. Biol.* **11**(9), 4431–4440.
11. Barrett, K., Taylor-Fishwick, D. A., Cope, A. P., Kissonerghis, A. M., Gray, P. W., Feldmann, M., and Foxwell, B. M. (1991). *Eur. J. Immunol.* **21**(7), 1649–1656.
12. Berg, M. M., Sternberg, D. W., Hempstead, B. L., and Chao, M. V. (1991). *Proc. Natl. Acad. Sci. U.S.A.* **88**(16), 7106–7110.
13. Beutler, B., and Cerami, A. (1988). *Annu. Rev. Biochem.* **57**(505), 505–518.
14. Bich-Thuy, L. t., Dukovich, M., Peffer, N. J., Fauci, A. S., Kehrl, J. H., and Greene, W. C. (1987). *J. Immunol.* **139**(5), 1550–1556.
15. Bomsztyk, K., Sims, J. E., Stanton, T. H., Slack, J., McMahan, C. J., Valentine, M. A., and Dower, S. K. (1989). *Proc. Natl. Acad. Sci. U.S.A.* **86**(20), 8034–8038.
16. Brakebusch, C., Nophar, Y., Kemper, O., Engelmann, H., and Wallach, D. (1992). *EMBO J.* **11**(3), 943–950.
17. Brockhaus, M., Schoenfeld, H. J., Schlaeger, E. J., Hunziker, W., Lesslauer, W., and Loetscher, H. (1990). *Proc. Natl. Acad. Sci. U.S.A.* **87**(8), 3127–3131.
18. Camerini, D., Walz, G., Loenen, W. A. M., Borst, J., and Seed, B. (1991). *J. Immunol.* **147**(9), 3165–3369.
19. Carter, D. B., Deibel, M. J., Dunn, C. J., Tomich, C. S., Laborde, A. L., Slightom, J. L., Berger, A. E., Bienkowski, M. J., Sun, F. F., and McEwan, R. N. (1990). *Nature (London)* **344**, 633–638.
20. Chun, M., and Hoffmann, M. K. (1987). *Lymphokine Res.* **6**(3), 161–167.
21. Churilla, A. M., Braciale, T. J., and Braciale, V. L. (1989). *J. Exp. Med.* **170**(1), 105–121.
22. Clark, E. A., and Shu, G. (1990). *J. Immunol.* **145**(5), 1400–1406.

23. Cleveland, J. L., Rapp, U. R., and Farrar, W. L. (1987). *J. Immunol.* **138**(10), 3495–3504.
24. Cordon-Cardo, C., Tapley, P., Jing, S. Q., Nanduri, V., O'Rourke, E., Lamballe, F., Kovary, K., Klein, R., Jones, K. R., and Reichardt, L. F. (1991) *Cell* **66**(1), 173–183.
25. Cosman, D., Wignall, K., Lewis, A., Alpert, A., McKereghan, K., Cerretti, D. P., Gillis, S., Dower, S., and Urdal, D. (1987). *In* "Molecular Cloning and Analysis of Lymphokines" (Webb and Goeddel, eds.). Academic Press, San Diego.
26. Cuturi, M. C., Murphy, M., Costa, G. M., Weinmann, R., Perussia, B., and Trinchieri, G. (1987). *J. Exp. Med.* **165**(6), 1581–1594.
27. Dawson, M. M. (1991). "Lymphokines and Interlcukins." Open Univ. Press. Milton Keynes.
28. Dibirdik, I., Langlie, M.-C., Ledbetter, J. A., Tuel-Ahlgren, L., Obuz, V., Waddick, K. G., Gajl-Peczalska, K., Schieven, G. L., and Uckun, F. M. (1991) *Blood* **78**(3), 564–570.
29. Donato, N. J., Gallick, G. E., Steck, P. A., and Rosenblum, M. G. (1989). *J. Biol. Chem.* **264**(34), 20,474–20,481.
30. Dower, S. K., and Sims, J. E. (1990). *Ann. Rheum. Dis.* **49**(1), 452–459.
31. Dukovich, M., Wano, Y., Bich-Thuy, L. t., Katz, P., Cullen, B. R., Kehrl, J. H., and Greene, W. C. (1987). *Nature (London)* **327**, 518–522.
32. Durkop, H., Latza, U., Hummel, M., Eitelbach, F., Seed, B., and Stein, H. (1992). *Cell.* **68**, 421–427.
33. Eardley, D. D., and Koshland, M. E. (1991). *Science* **251**, 78–81.
34. Eck, M. J., Ultsch, M., Rinderknecht, E., de Vos, A. M., and Sprang, S. R. (1992). *J. Biol. Chem.* **267**(4), 2119–2122.
35. Engelmann, H., Holtmann, H., Brakebusch, C., Avni, Y. S., Sarov, I., Nophar, Y., Hadas, E., Leitner, O., and Wallach, D. (1990). *J. Biol. Chem.* **265**(24), 14,497–14,504.
36. Engelmann, H., Novick, D., and Wallach, D. (1990). *J. Biol. Chem.* **265**(3), 1531–1536.
37. Espevik, T., Brockhaus, M., Loetscher, H., Nonstad, U., and Shalaby, R. (1990). *J. Exp. Med.* **171**(2), 415–426.
38. Essner, R., Rhoades, K., McBride, W. H., Morton, D. L., and Economou, J. S. (1989). *J. Immunol.* **142**(11), 3857–3861.
39. Evans, S. W., Beckner, S. K., and Farra, W. L. (1987). *Nature (London)* **325**, 166–168. [Published erratum appears in *Nature (London)* (1987) **327**, 467].
40. Fernandez-Botran, R., and Vitetta, E. S. (1991). *J. Exp. Med.* **174**(3), 673–681.
41. Ferris, D. K., Willette-Brown, J., Ortaldo, J. R., and Farrar, W. L. (1989). *J. Immunol.* **143**(3), 870–876.
42. Finney, M., Guy, G. R., Michell, R. H., Gordon, J., Dugas, B., Rigley, K. P., and Callard, R. E. (1990). *Eur. J. Immunol.* **20**(1), 151–156.
43. Fountoulakis, M., Juranville, J. F., Maris, A., Ozmen, L., and Garotta, G. (1990). *J. Biol. Chem.* **265**(32), 19,758–19,767.
44. Foxwell, B. M., Woerly, G., and Ryffel, B. (1989). *Eur. J. Immunol.* **19**(9); 1637–1641.
45. Foxwell, B. M. J., Taylor-Fishwick, D. A., Simon, J. L., Page, T. H., and Londei, M. (1992). *Int. Immunol.* **4**(2), 277–282.
46. Fukunaga, R., Ishizaka-Ikeda, E., and Nagata, S. (1990). *J. Biol. Chem.* **265**(23), 14,008–14,015.
47. Fukunaga, R., Ishizaka-Ikeda, E., Seto, Y., and Nagata, S. (1990). *Cell* **61**(2), 341–350.
48. Galizzi, J.-P., Zuber, C. E., Harada, N., Gorman, D. M., Djossou, O., Kastelein, R., Banchereau, J., Howard, M., and Miyajima, A. (1990). *Int. Immunol.* **2**(7), 699–675.
49. Galizzi, J.-P., Cabrillat, H., Rousset, F., Menetrier, C., and Banchereau, J. (1988). *J. Immunol.* **141**(6), 1982–1988.
50. Gearing, D. P., Comeau, M. R., Friend, D. J., Gimpel, S. D., Thut, C. J., McGourty, J., Brasher, K. K., King, J. A., Gillis, S., Mosley, B., Ziegler, S. F., and Cosman, D. (1992). **255**, 1434–1437.
51. Gearing, D. P., King, J. A., Gough, N. M., and Nicola, N. A. (1989). *EMBO J.* **8**(12), 3667–3676.

52. Goeddel, D. V., Aggarwal, B. B., Gray, P. W., Leung, D. W., Nedwin, G. E., Palladino, M. A., Patton, J. S., Pennica, D., Shepard, H. M., and Sugarman, B. J. (1986). *Cold Spring Harb. Symp. Quant. Biol.* **1,** 597–609.

53. Goodwin, R. G., Friend, D., Ziegler, S. F., Jerzy, R., Falk, B. A., Gimpel, S., Cosman, D., Dower, S. K., March, C. J., and Namen, A. E. (1990). *Cell* **60**(6), 941–951.

54. Gordon, J., Katira, A., Strain, A. J., and Gillis, S. (1991). *Eur. J. Immunol.* **21**(8), 1917–1922.

55. Gorman, D. M., Itoh, N., Kitamura, T., Schreurs, J., Yonehara, S., Yahara, I., Arai, K., and Miyajima, A. (1990). *Proc. Natl. Acad. Sci. U.S.A.* **87**(14), 5459–5463.

56. Graves, J. D., Downward, J., Izquierdo-Pastor, M., Rayter, S., Warne, P. H., and Cantrell, D. A. (1992). Submitted for publication.

57. Gray, P. W., Barrett, K., Chantry, D., Turner, M., and Feldmann, M. (1990). *Proc. Natl. Acad. Sci. U.S.A.* **87**(19), 7380–7384.

58. Gray, P. W., Leong, S., Fennie, E. H., Farrar, M. A., Pingel, J. T., Fernandez, L. J., and Schreiber, R. D. (1989). *Proc. Natl. Acad. Sci. U.S.A.* **86**(21), 8497–8501.

59. Green, S. H., Rydel, R. E., Connolly, J. L., and Greene, L. A. (1986). *J. Cell Biol.* **102**(3), 830–843.

60. Hama, T., Huang, K. P., and Guroff, G. (1986). *Proc. Natl. Acad. Sci. U.S.A.* **83**(8), 2353–2357.

61. Harada, N., Castle, B. E., Gorman, D. M., Itoh, N., Schreurs, J., Barrett, R. L., Howard, M., and Miyajima, A. (1990). *Proc. Natl. Acad. Sci. U.S.A.* **87**(3), 857–861.

62. Hatakeyama, M., Kono, T., Kobayashi, N., Kawahara, A., Levin, S. D., Perlmutter, R. M., and Taniguchi, T. (1991). *Science* **252,** 1523–1528.

63. Hatakeyama, M., Tsudo, M., Minamoto, S., Kono, T., Doi, T., Miyata, T., Miyasaka, M., and Taniguchi, T. (1989). *Science* **244, 551–556.**

64. Hempstead, B. L., Martin-Zanca, D., Kaplan, D. R., Parada, L. F., and Chao, M. V. (1991). *Nature* (*London*) **350,** 678–683.

65. Henney, C. S. (1989). *Immunol. Today* **10**(5), 170–173.

66. Herrmann, T., and Diamantstein, T. (1987). *Immunobiology* **175**(3), 145–158.

67. Hibi, M., Murakami, M., Saito, M., Hirano, T., Taga, T., and Kishimoto, T. (1990). *Cell* **63**(6), 1149–1157.

68. Hibino, Y., Kumar, C. S., Mariano, T. M., Lai, D., and Pestka, S. (1992). *J. Biol. Chem.* **267**(6), 3741–3749.

69. Hibino, Y., Mariano, T. M., Kumar, C. S., Kozak, C. A., and Pestka, S. (1991). *J. Biol. Chem.* **266**(11), 6948–6951.

70. Hohmann, H. P., Remy, R., Brockhaus, M., and Van Loon, A. P. (1989). *J. Biol. Chem.* **264**(25), 14,927–14,934.

71. Howells, G., Pham, P., Taylor, D., Foxwell, B., and Feldmann, M. (1991). *Eur. J. Immunol.* **21**(1), 97–101.

72. Idzerda, R. L., March, C. J., Mosley, B., Lyman, S. D., VandenBos, T., Gimpel, S. D., Din, W. S., Grabstein, K. H., Widmer, M. B., and Park, L. S. (1990). *J. Exp. Med.* **171**(3), 861–873.

73. Imamura, K., Sherman, M. L., Spriggs, D., and Kufe, D. (1988). *J. Biol. Chem.* **263**(21), 10,247–10,253.

74. Inui, S., Kaisho, T., Kikutani, H., Stamenkovic, I., Seed, B., Clark, E. A., and Kishimoto, T. (1990). *Eur. J. Immunol.* **20**(8), 1747–1753.

75. Isfort, R. J., and Ihle, J. N. (1990). *Growth Factors* **2,**. 213–220.

76. Isfort, R. J., Stevens, D., May, W. S., and Ihle, J. N. (1988). *Proc. Natl. Acad. Sci. U.S.A.* **85**(21), 7982–7986.

77. Ishii, T., Takeshita, T., Numata, N., and Sugamura, K. (1988). *J. Immunol.* **141**(1), 174–179.

78. Itoh, N., Yonehara, S., Ishii, A., Yonehara, M., Mizushima, S., Sameshima, M., Hase, A., Seto, Y., and Nagata, S. (1991). *Cell* **66**(2), 233–243.

79. Itoh, N., Yonehara, S., Schreurs, J., Gorman, D. M., Maruyama, K., Ishii, A., Yahara, I., Arai, K., and Miyajima, A. (1990). *Science* **247**, 324–327.

80. Izquierdo, M., Downward, J., Otani, H., Leonard, W. J., and Cantrell, D. A. (1992). *Eur. J. Immunol.* **22**, 817–821.

81. Johnson, D., Lanahan, A., Buck, C. R., Sehgal, A., Morgan, C., Mercer, E., Bothwell, M., and Chao, M. (1986). *Cell* **47**(4), 545–554.

82. Jones, E. Y., Stuart, D. I., and Walker, N. P. (1989). *Nature (London)* **338**, 225–228.

83. Jung, V., Jones, C., Kumar, C. S., Stefanos, S., O'Connell, S., and Pestka, S. (1990). *J. Biol. Chem.* **265**(4), 1827–1830.

84. Kaplan, D. R., Martin-Zanca, D., and Parada, L. F. (1991). *Nature (London)* **350**, 158–160.

85. Keegan, A. D., Beckmann, M. P., Park, L. S., and Paul, W. E. (1991). *J. Immunol.* **146**(7), 2272–2279.

86. Kitamura, T., Hayashida, K., Sakamaki, K., Yokota, T., Arai, K.-i., and Miyajima, A. (1991). *Proc. Natl. Acad. Sci. U.S.A.* **88**(12), 5082–5086.

87. Kitamura, T., Sato, N., Arai, K.-i., and Miyajima, A. (1991). *Cell* **66**(6), 1165–1174.

88. Klein, R., Jing, S. Q., Nanduri, V., O'Rourke, E., and Barbacid, M. (1991). *Cell* **65**(1), 189–197.

89. Klein, R., Nanduri, V., Jing, S. A., Lamballe, F., Tapley, P., Bryant, S., Cordon-Cardo, C., Jones, K. R., Reichardt, L. F., and Barbacid, M. (1991). *Cell* **66**(2), 395–403.

90. Kohno, M., Nishizawa, N., Tsujimoto, M., and Nomoto, H. (1990). *Biochem. J.* **267**(1), 91–98.

91. Kwon, B. S., and Weissman, S. M. (1989). *Proc. Natl. Acad. Sci. U.S.A.* **86**(6), 1963–1967.

92. Larrick, J. W., and Wright, S. C. (1990). *FASEB J.* **4**(14), 3215–3223.

93. Larsen, A., Davis, T., Curtis, B. M., Gimpel, S., Sims, J. E., Cosman, D., Park, L., Sorensen, E., March, C. J., and Smith, C. A. (1990). *J. Exp. Med.* **172**(6), 1559–1570.

94. Leonard, W. J. (1987). *In* "Molecular Cloning and Analysis of Lymphokines" (Z. Webb and D. V. Goeddel, eds.). Academic, Press, San Diego.

95. Loetscher, H., Pan, Y. C., Lahm, H. W., Gentz, R., Brockhaus, M., Tabuchi, H., and Lesslauer, W. (1990). *Cell* **61**(2), 351–359.

96. Longmore, G. D., and Lodish, H. F. (1991). *Cell* **67**, 1089–1102.

97. Lowenthal, J. W., and Greene, W. C. (1987). *J. Exp. Med.* **166**(4), 1156–1161.

98. Mallett, S., Fossum, S., and Barclay, A. N. (1990). *EMBO J.* **9**(4), 1063–1068.

99. Merida, I., and Gaulton, G. N. (1990). *J. Biol. Chem.* **265**(10), 5690–5694.

100. Miller, J., Mallek, T. R., Shevach, E. M., and Germain, R. N. (1987). *In* "Molecular Cloning and Analysis of Lymphokines" (Webb and Goeddel, eds.). Academic Press, San Diego.

101. Mills, G. B., Girard, P., Grinstein, S., and Gelfand, E. W. (1988). *Cell* **55**(1), 91–100.

102. Mizel, S. B. (1990). *Immunol. Today* **11**, 390–391.

103. Mosley, B., Beckmann, M. P., March, C. J., Idzerda, R. L., Gimpel, S. D., VandenBos, T., Friend, D., Alpert, A., Anderson, D., and Jackson, J. (1989). *Cell* **59**(2), 335–348.

104. Murakami, M., Narazaki, M., Hibi, M., Yawata, H., Yasukawa, K., Hamaguchi, M., Taga, T., and Kishimoto, T. (1991). *Proc. Natl. Acad. Sci. U.S.A.* **88**, 11,349–11,353.

105. Murata, Y., Yamaguchi, N., Hitoshi, Y., Tonimaga, A., and Takatsu, K. (1990). *Biochem. Biophys. Res. Commun.* **173**, 1102–1108.

106. Nagata, S., Tsuchiya, M., Asano, S., Kaziro, Y., Yamazaki, T., Yamamoto, O., Hirata, Y., Kubota, N., Oheda, M., and Nomura, H., (1986). *Nature (London)* **319**, 415–418.

107. Nedwin, G. E., Svedersky, L. P., Bringman, T. S., Palladino, M. J., and Goeddel, D. V. (1985). *J. Immunol.* **135**(4), 2492–2497.

108. Novick, D., Engelmann, H., Wallach, D., and Rubinstein, M. (1989). *J. Exp. Med.* **170**(4), 1409–1414.

109. O'Neill, L. J., Bird, T. A., and Saklatvala, J. (1990). *Immunol. Today* **11**, 392–394.

110. Olsson, I., Lantz, M., Nilsson, E., Peetre, C., Thysell, H., Grubb, A., and Adolf, G. (1989). *Eur. J. Haematol.* **42**(3), 270–275.

111. Oppenheim, J. J., Kovacs, E. J., Matsushima, K., and Durum, S. K. (1986). *Immunol. Today* **7**, 45–56.

112. Ostrowski, J., Meier, K. E., Stanton, T. H., Smith, L. L., and Bomsztyk, K. (1988). *J. Biol. Chem.* **263**(27), 13,786–13,790.

113. Park, L. S., Friend, D., Price, V., Anderson, D., Singer, J., Prickett, K. S., and Urdal, D. L. (1989). *J. Biol. Chem.* **264**(10), 5420–5427.

114. Park, L. S., Friend, D. J., Schmierer, A. E., Dower, S. K., and Namen, A. E. (1990). *J. Exp. Med.* **171**(4), 1073–1089.

115. Paul, N. L., and Ruddle, N. H. (1988). *Annu. Rev. Immunol.* **6**, 407–438.

116. Porteu, F., Brockhaus, M., Wallach, D., Engelmann, H., and Nathan, C. F. (1991). *J. Biol. Chem.* **266**(28), 18,846–18,853.

117. Remillard, B., Petrillo, R., Maslinski, W., Tsudo, M., Strom, T. B., Cantley, L., and Varticovski, L. (1991). *J. Biol. Chem.* **266**(22), 14,167–14,170.

118. Rigley, K. P., Thurstan, S. M., and Callard, R. E. (1991). *Int. Immunol.* **3**(2), 197–203.

119. Robb, R. J., and Greene, W. C. (1987). *J. Exp. Med.* **165**(4), 1201–1206.

120. Robb, R. J., Greene, W. C., and Rusk, C. M. (1984). *J. Exp. Med.* **160**, 1126–1146.

121. Robb, R. J., Rusk, C. M., Yodoi, J., and Greene, W. C. (1987). *Proc. Natl. Acad. Sci. U.S.A.* **84**(7), 2002–2006.

122. Roifman, C. M., Wang, G., Freedman, M., and Pan, Z. (1992). *J. Immunol.* **148**(4), 1136–1142.

123. Rubin, B. Y., Anderson, S. L., Sullivan, S. A., Williamson, B. D., Carswell, E. A., and Old, L. J. (1986). *J. Exp. Med.* **164**(4), 1350–1355.

124. Rubin, L. A., Kurman, C. C., Fritz, M. E., Biddison, W. E., Boutin, B., Yarchoan, R., and Nelson, D. L. (1985). *J. Immunol.* **135**(5), 3172–3177.

125. Saltzman, E. M., Thom, R. R., and Casnellie, J. E. (1988). *J. Biol. Chem.* **263**(15), 6956–6959.

126. Saragovi, H., and Malek, T. R. (1988). *J. Immunol.* **141**(2), 476–482.

127. Saragovi, H., and Malek, T. R. (1990). *Proc. Natl. Acad. Sci. U.S.A.* **87**(1), 11–15.

128. Satoh, T., Nakafuku, M., Miyajima, A., and Kaziro, Y. (1991). *Proc. Natl. Acad. Sci. U.S.A.* **88**(8), 3314–3318.

129. Schall, T. J., Lewis, M., Koller, K. J., Lee, A., Rice, G. C., Wong, G. H., Gatanaga, T., Granger, G. A., Lentz, R., Raab, H., Kohr, W. J., and Goedel, D. V. (1990). *Cell* **61**(2), 361–370.

130. Schutze, S., Scheurich, P., Pfizenmaier, K., and Kronke, M. (1989). *J. Biol. Chem.* **264**(6), 3562–3567.

131. Seckinger, P., Isaaz, S., and Dayer, J. M. (1989). *J. Biol. Chem.* **264**(20), 11,966–11,973.

132. Sharon, M., Gnarra, J. R., and Leonard, W. J. (1989). *J. Immunol.* **143**(8), 2530–2533.

133. Sharon, M., Gnarra, J. R., and Leonard, W. J. (1990). *Proc. Natl. Acad. Sci. U.S.A.* **87**(12), 4869–4873.

134. Sharon, M., Klausner, R. D., Cullen, B. R., Chizzonite, R., and Leonard, W. J. (1986) *Science* **234**, 859–863.

135. Siegel, J. P., Sharon, M., Smith, P. L., and Leonard, W. J. (1987). *Science* **238**, 75–78.

136. Sims, J. E., March, C. J., Cosman, D., Widmer, M. B., MacDonald, H. R., McMahan, C. J., Grubin, C. E., Wignall, J. M., Jackson, J. L., and Call, S. M. (1988). *Science* **241**, 585–589.

137. Smith, C. A., Davis, T., Anderson, D., Solam, L., Beckmann, M. P., Jerzy, R., Dower, S. K., Cosman, D., and Goodwin, R. G. (1990). *Science* **248**, 1019–1023.

138. Smith, C. A., Davis, T., Wignall, J. M., Din, W. S., Farrah, T., Upton, C., McFadden, G., and Goodwin, R. G. (1991). *Biochem. Biophys. Res. Commun.* **176**, 335–342.

139. Smith, K. A. (1988). *Adv. Immunol.* **42**, 165–179.

140. Smith, K. A. (1988). *Science* **240**, 1169–1176.

141. Smith, M. R., Munger, W. E., Kung, H. F., Takacs, L., and Durum, S. K. (1990). *J. Immunol.* **144**(1), 162–169.

142. Smith, R. A., and Baglioni, C. (1987). *J. Biol. Chem.* **262**(15), 6951–6954.

143. Smith, R. A., and Baglioni, C. (1989). *J. Biol. Chem.* **264**(25), 14,646–14,652.

144. Spriggs, D. R., Imamura, K., Rodriguez, C., Sariban, E., and Kufe, D. W. (1988). *J. Clin. Invest.* **81**(2), 455–460.

145. Stamenkovic, I., Clark, E. A., and Seed, B. (1989). *EMBO J.* **8**(5), 1403–1410.

146. Stauber, G. B., Aiyer, R. A., and Aggarwal, B. B. (1988). *J. Biol. Chem.* **263**(35), 19,098–19,104.

147. Sung, S. S., Bjorndahl, J. M., Wang, C. Y., Kao, H. T., and Fu, S. M. (1988). *J. Exp. Med.* **167**(3), 937–953.

148. Taga, T., Hibi, M., Hirata, Y., Yamasaki, K., Yasukawa, K., Matsuda, T., Hirano, T., and Kishimoto, T. (1989). *Cell* **58**(3), 573–581.

149. Takaki, S., Tominaga, A., Hitoshi, Y., Mita, S., Sonoda, E., Yamaguchi, N., and Takatsu, K. (1990). *EMBO J.* **9**(13), 4367–4374.

150. Tartaglia, L. A., and Goeddel, D. V. (1992). *J. Biol. Chem.* **267**(7), 4304–4307.

151. Tartaglia, L. A., Weber, R. F., Figari, I. S., Reynolds, C., Palladino, M. A., Jr., and Goeddel, D. V. (1991). *Proc. Natl. Acad. Sci. U.S.A.* **88**, 9292–9296.

152. Tavernier, J., Devos, R., Cornelis, S., Tuypens, T., Van der Heyden, J., Fiers, W., and Plaetinck, G. (1991). *Cell* **66**(6), 1175–1184.

153. Teshigawara, K., Wang, H.-M., Kato, K., and Smith, K. A. (1987). *J. Exp. Med.* **165**(1), 223–238.

154. Tigges, M. A., Casey, L. S., and Koshland, M. E. (1989). *Science* **243**, 781–786.

155. Tsudo, M., Karasuyama, H., Kitamura, F., Tanaka, T., Kubo, S., Yamamura, Y., Tamatani, T., Hatakeyama, M., Taniguchi, T., and Miyasaka, M. (1990). *J. Immunol.* **145**(2), 599–606.

156. Tsudo, M., Kozak, R. W., Goldman, C. K., and Waldmann, T. A. (1987). *Proc. Natl. Acad. Sci. U.S.A.* **84**(12), 4215–4218.

157. Turner, M., Londei, M., and Feldmann, M. (1987). *Eur. J. Immunol.* **17**(12), 1807–1814.

158. Uckun, F. M., Dibirdik, I., Smith, R., Tuel-Ahlgren, L., Langlie, M.-C., and Schieven, G. L. (1991). *Proc. Natl. Acad. Sci. U.S.A.* **88**(9), 3589–3593.

159. Uckun, F. M., Schieven, G. L., Dibirdik, I., Langlie, M.-C., Tuel-Ahlgren, L., and Ledbetter, J. A. (1991). *J. Biol. Chem.* **266**(26), 17,478–17,485.

160. Uckun, F. M., Tuel-Ahlgren, L., Obuz, V., Smith, R., Dibirdik, I., Hanson, M., and Langlie, M.-C. (1991). *Proc. Natl. Acad. Sci. U.S.A.* **88**(14), 6323–6327.

161. Upton, C., DeLange, A. M., and McFadden, G. (1987). *Virology* **160**(1), 20–30.

162. Valentine, M. A., Widmer, M. B., Ledbetter, J. A., Pinault, F., Voice, R., Clark, E. A., Gallis, B., and Brautigan, D. L. (1991). *Eur. J. Immunol.* **21**(4), 913–919.

163. Valge, V. E., Wong, J. G., Datlof, B. M., Sinskey, A. J., and Rao, A. (1988). *Cell* **55**(1), 101–112.

164. Venkatakrishnan, G., McKinnon, C. A., Pilapil, C. G., Wolf, D. E., and Ross, A. H. (1991). *Biochemistry* **30**(11), 2748–2753.

165. Waldmann, T. A. (1991). *J. Biol. Chem.* **266**(5), 2681–2684.

166. Wang, H. M., and Smith, K. A. (1987). *J. Exp. Med.* **166**(4), 1055–1069.

167. Weiss, L., Haeffner-Cavaillon, N., Laude, M., Cavaillon, J. M., and Kazatchkine, M. D. (1989). *Eur. J. Immunol.* **19**(7), 1347–1350.

168. Yagita, H., Nakata, M., Azuma, A., Nitta, T., Takeshita, T., Sugamura, K., and Okumura, K. (1989). *J. Exp. Med.* **170**(4), 1445–1450.

169. Yamasaki, K., Taga, T., Hirata, Y., Yawata, H., Kawanishi, Y., Seed, B., Taniguchi, T., Hirano, T., and Kishimoto, T. (1988). *Science* **241** 825–828.

170. Zhang, Y. H., Lin, J.X., Yip, Y. K., and Vilcek, J. (1988). *Proc. Natl. Acad. Sci. U.S.A.* **85**(18), 6802–6805.

171. Zmuidzinas, A., Mamon, H. J., Roberts, T. M., and Smith, K. A. (1991). *Mol. Cell. Biol.* **11**(5), 2794–2803.

Pharmacokinetic Parameters and Biodistribution of Soluble Cytokine Receptors

Cindy A. Jacobs, M. Patricia Beckmann, Ken Mohler, Charles R. Maliszewski, William C. Fanslow, and David H. Lynch

Immunex Corporation
Seattle, Washington 98101

I. INTRODUCTION

Cytokines are hormonelike regulatory molecules of the immune system. Their many regulatory roles include controlling cellular and humoral immune responses, chemotaxis, antitumor immune responses, hematopoiesis, inflammation, and many other functions (Smith, 1990; Paul, 1989). Insufficient production of such cytokines can lead to immune-deficient states whereas continued uninhibited production may lead to autoimmunity, allergy, or other chronic inflammatory states. *In vivo,* cytokines do not usually act alone but in combination with other cytokines and stimuli. Combinations

International Review of Experimental Pathology, Volume 34B

of cytokines may be synergistic or antagonistic in their actions, which complicates investigating their mechanistic roles in the immune system.

Cytokines mediate their functions by binding to their specific membrane-associated receptors. These cytokine receptors are integral membrane proteins composed of an extracellular ligand-binding region, a membrane-spanning region, and an intracellular region that is activated by cytokine binding and hence delivers a signal. A number of cytokine receptors have also been demonstrated to exist in soluble form in the biological fluids of both animals and humans (Fanslow *et al.,* 1990a; Fernandez-Botran, 1991). Some of these soluble receptors are naturally occurring, secreted products and others are thought to be proteolytically cleaved from the intact membrane form. Although many cytokine receptors have not yet been detected as naturally occurring soluble products, molecular cloning and engineering have allowed isolation and truncation of some cDNAs encoding the intact membrane form of a receptor to produce a soluble form consisting of only the extracellular ligand-binding region (Dower *et al.,* 1989).

The existence of soluble cytokine receptors has immunoregulatory implications and significant potential for therapeutic use as very specific anticytokine agents and as probes for examining the roles of their respective cytokines in the immune system (Maliszewski and Fanslow, 1990). As the affinity of most soluble receptors for their ligands is usually comparable to that of the membrane-associated receptor, soluble receptors can compete with membrane-associated receptors for binding of free cytokines and thus act as very specific cytokine inhibitors. Administration of a soluble receptor would therefore inhibit the biological activity of a cytokine by binding the free cytokine and preventing it from binding and activating the membrane-associated receptor. Preclinical investigation into the pharmacokinetic properties and biodistribution patterns of the various soluble cytokine receptors allows an estimation of their serum half-life, the frequency of administration as potential therapeutic products, and dosage requirements for planning clinical trials. In addition, the preclinical biodistribution patterns of organ accumulation or clearance of the receptor allow for more precise monitoring of safety parameters. Differences in the pharmacokinetic parameters have been observed for each soluble receptor, with biodistribution patterns specific for that receptor.

II. METHODS OF PHARMACOKINETIC AND BIODISTRIBUTION ANALYSIS

A. Study Design

Radiolabeled soluble receptors were evaluated as monomers and in some cases as dimers in the form of fusion proteins. Because interleukin-1 receptor

(IL-1R) and interleukin-4 receptor (IL-4R) are species specific, monomeric forms of soluble mouse IL-1R and mouse IL-4R were used in the studies (Dower *et al.,* 1989; Jacobs *et al.,* 1991b). Both IL-1R and the IL-4R are produced in HeLa cells. In addition, an Il-4R fusion protein containing two soluble mouse IL-4R monomers on a mouse IgG_{2b} Fc structure was evaluated. Various forms of soluble human tumor necrosis factor receptor (TNF-R) were also analyzed in mice because human TNF-R can bind either murine TNF-α or TNF-β. Two forms of monomeric TNF-R were evaluated: an unglycosylated form produced by an *Escherichia coli* expression system and a glycosylated form produced by a CHO expression system. A TNF-R fusion protein containing two soluble human TNF-R monomers on a human IgG_1 Fc structure was also evaluated. Both fusion proteins were produced in BHK cells.

Soluble receptors were radiolabeled with ^{125}I by the Enzymobead technique (Biorad, Richmond, California) and stored in phosphate-buffered saline (PBS) containing 0.01% mouse serum albumin. Radiolabeling was performed within 7–10 days prior to pharmacokinetic studies and receptors were analyzed for cytokine binding to assure that loss of receptor-binding ability to the specific cytokine ligand had not occurred.

Experiments were performed using BALB/c mice (Jackson Laboratory, Bar Harbor, Maine), 7–10 weeks of age, weighing 17 to 21 g. The mice were maintained at Immunex Corporation in a specific pathogen-free animal facility for a minimum of 1–2 weeks prior to experiments and fed *ad libitum.* The radiolabeled receptors were injected intravenously (i.v.) via the lateral tail vein, intraperitoneally (i.p.), or subcutaneously (s.c.) at the nape of the neck in a total volume of 150 μl. At various time points ranging from 2 min to 48 hr, groups of mice (three mice per group) were bled by cardiac puncture and were sacrificed. Blood samples were heparinized, weighed, and the radioactivity was determined using a Packard Cobra Autogamma Scintillation counter (Packard Instruments, Laguna Hills, California). Plasma was then isolated from the aliquot of blood and the actual TCA-precipitable counts were determined for blood samples. Five additional tissues (liver, kidney, spleen, lung, and heart) were collected, weighed, and the radioactivity determined as described above. All blood and tissue samples were represented as a percentage of the injected dose per gram of the collected tissue (% ID/g) (Gennuso *et al.,* 1989). The actual amounts of soluble receptor per gram of tissue (ng/g or μg/g) and per organ weight were calculated using a percentage of organ weights relative to the whole body weight of the mice. Data are represented as the mean $\pm$ standard error (SE) per time point.

B. Pharmacokinetic Data Analysis

Pharmacokinetic parameters were determined from the blood concentration–time profiles for each route of administration and each soluble receptor preparation (Gustavson *et al.,* 1989). Pharmacokinetic parameters for liver and kidney were estimated using the tissue concentration–time profiles for each route of administration. The apparent elimination rate constant (K) and half-life ($T_{1/2}$) were calculated using a pharmacokinetics half-life program on a RS/1 computer system. The log linear portion of the blood or tissue concentration–time curve was used to calculate K. The $T_{1/2}$ was determined as $T_{1/2} = \ln 2/K$. Half-life values are presented as $T_{1/2} \pm$ SE, where SE indicates the error in fitting the log linear line to the data points in calculating the K value. For the i.v. route of administration, the distribution ($T_{1/2\alpha}$) and elimination ($T_{1/2\beta}$) half-lives were calculated using a biphasic pharmacokinetics program relating respective log linear concentration–time curves to specific K and $T_{1/2}$ values. The area under the blood or tissue concentration–time curve (AUC) from time 0 to infinite time was determined by conventional trapezoidal summation and extrapolation. The maximum serum concentration (C_{max}) and the time of maximum serum concentration (T_{max}) were read directly from the plotted data. To evaluate soluble receptor biodistribution levels in tissue over time, cumulative tissue distribution values for all tissues were determined by AUC analysis. Cumulative tissue biodistribution values for the amounts of soluble receptors per gram of tissue as well as per actual organ weights are also calculated.

III. SOLUBLE IL-1 RECEPTOR

A. Blood Clearance

The clearance of intravenously administered soluble IL-1R (sIL-1R) corresponds to two phases described by two exponentials: an initial distribution half-life ($T_{1/2\alpha}$) and a second elimination half-life ($T_{1/2\beta}$). The blood distribution half-life ($T_{1/2\alpha}$) for a single i.v. bolus injection of sIL-1R was 16 ± 4 min (Table I). Approximately 23% of the injected dose was cleared during this phase and was 90% completed within 53 minutes (3.3 half-lives = 90%). During this period, the initial distribution was mainly to liver and kidneys; however, the C_{max} for blood was still two- to threefold greater than the C_{max} for either liver or kidneys. The blood elimination half-life ($T_{1/2\beta}$) of sIL-1R was 6.3 ± 1.3 hr with the remaining 77% of the initial injected dose eliminated in 32 hr (5 half-lives). Elimination was mediated by both liver and kidneys, which had $T_{1/2\beta}$ values of 2.0 and 3.2 hr, respectively (Table I).

When sIL-1R was administered by i.p. or s.c. routes as compared with i.v. administration, the blood kinetics showed delayed T_{max} values (120 and 240 min, respectively) and corresponding decreases in the C_{max} values (Table I). The $T_{1/2\beta}$ value for i.p. administration (5.0 ± 0.8 hr) was similar to i.v. administration whereas the s.c. administration was prolonged to 9.5 ± 1.3 hr.

Table I. sIL-1R Pharmacokinetic Parameters

Parameter	Intravenous	Intraperitoneal	Subcutaneous
		Route of administration[a]	
Blood kinetics			
C_{max}	178 ng/ml	32 ng/ml	14 ng/ml
T_{max}	1 min	120 min	240 min
$T_{1/2\alpha}$	16 ± 4 min	—	—
$T_{1/2\beta}$	6.3 ± 1.3 hr	5.0 ± 0.8 hr	9.5 ± 1.3 hr
Tissue kinetics			
Kidney			
C_{max}	50 ng/g	28 ng/g	6 ng/g
T_{max}	5 min	120 min	60 min
$T_{1/2\beta}$	3.2 ± 0.7 hr	4.0 ± 0.8 hr	7.7 ± 0.8 hr
Liver			
C_{max}	79 ng/g	19 ng/g	7 ng/g
T_{max}	5 min	60 min	120 min
$T_{1/2\beta}$	2.0 ± 0.6 hr	3.8 ± 0.8 hr	8.4 ± 1.5 hr

[a] Mice were injected with 340 ng (i.v.) or 240 ng (i.p. and s.c.) of TCA-precipitable, ^{125}I-labeled sIL-1R at time 0.

B. Tissue Distribution

On a per gram basis or per organ basis, estimating the blood volume to be 8% of body weight, the highest cumulative levels of sIL-1R when administered i.v. occurred in the blood (Table II). On a per gram basis, kidney, liver, and lung were major sites for cumulative sIL-1R tissue levels. However, on a per organ basis, the liver was the major site of accumulation, followed by kidney. Spleen, lung, and heart showed minimal levels of accumulation on a per organ basis. Although liver was the major site of accumulation and most likely elimination, only 17% of the sIL-1R observed in the blood was distributed to the liver.

IV. SOLUBLE IL-4 RECEPTOR

A. Blood Clearance

The clearance of intravenously administered sIL-4R also showed a biphasic exponential curve. The $T_{1/2\alpha}$ for a single bolus i.v. injection of sIL-4R was 9 min (Table III). Approximately 75% of the injected dose was cleared during this phase and was 90% completed within 30 min. During this phase, liver was the primary site of distribution, having a C_{max} comparable with that of blood levels. Kidneys were the second site of distribution, with a C_{max}

Table II. Cumulative Tissue Biodistribution for Soluble Cytokine Receptors

| | Type of soluble cytokine receptor administered[a] | | | | | |
| | sIL-1R | | sIL-4R | | sTNFR | |
Organ	μg/g	μg/organ	μg/g	μg/organ	μg/g	μg/organ
Blood	45	77	91	116	15	25
Kidney	14	5	65	16	28	9
Liver	13	13	65	50	6	6
Spleen	7	1	50	4	7	1
Lung	13	2	74	8	12	2
Heart	9	1	39	4	7	1

[a] Cumulative tissue biodistributions were determined by calculating the area under the blood (or tissue) concentration–time curve from time 0 to infinite time. The actual amount of soluble receptor per gram of tissue (μg/g) or per organ (μg/organ) was calculated for each receptor, given that 340 ng sIL-1R, 1.1 μg sIL-4R, and 300 ng sTNF-R (CHO) were administered per mouse by i.v. injection.

value approximately half of that detected in liver. The elimination phase had a $T_{1/2\beta}$ of 2.3 ± 0.8 hr with the remaining 25% of the injected dose eliminated in 11 hr. Rapid elimination was mediated by the liver with a $\tilde{T}_{1/2\beta}$ of 0.4 hr and slower elimination was mediated by kidneys ($T_{1/2\beta}$ of 1.2 hr).

Table III. sIL-4R Pharmacokinetic Parameters

| | Route of Administration[a] | | |
Parameter	Intravenous	Intraperitoneal	Subcutaneous
Blood kinetics			
C_{max}	1.2 μg/ml	0.19 μg/ml	0.21 μg/ml
T_{max}	2 min	60 min	60 min
$T_{1/2\alpha}$	9 ± 1 min	—	—
$T_{1/2\beta}$	2.3 ± 0.8 hr	4.2 ± 2.1 hr	6.2 ± 2.0 hr
Tissue kinetics			
Kidney			
C_{max}	0.68 μg/g	0.26 μg/g	0.18 μg/g
T_{max}	3 min	15 min	60 min
$T_{1/2\beta}$	1.2 ± 0.4 hr	5.5 ± 1.7 hr	4.7 ± 0.8 hr
Liver			
C_{max}	1.15 μg/g	0.15 μg/g	0.10 μg/g
T_{max}	5 min	15 min	120 min
$T_{1/2\beta}$	0.4 ± 0.1 hr	4.4 ± 0.8 hr	4.6 ± 1.0 hr

[a] Mice were injected with 1.1 μg of TCA-precipitable, ^{125}I-labeled sIL-4R by i.v., i.p., or s.c. injections at time 0.

When sIL-4R was administered by either i.p. or s.c. routes, the blood kinetics showed delayed $T_{\max}$ values, decreased $C_{\max}$ values, and prolonged $T_{1/2\beta}$ values compared to i.v. administration (Table III). The $T_{\max}$ values for i.p. and s.c. sIL-4R were 60 min compared to 2 min for i.v. injection. The $C_{\max}$ values were similar for both i.p. and s.c. routes and approximately sixfold lower than the $C_{\max}$ value observed following i.v. injection. The $T_{1/2\beta}$ values for i.p. and s.c. routes were 4.2 and 6.2 hr, respectively. Distribution of sIL-4R to tissues was generally lower in concentration and prolonged over time, especially for liver, when sIL-4R was administered by s.c. injection.

B. Tissue Distribution

Cumulative tissue distribution levels indicated that significant amounts of sIL-4R were detectable in the blood. On a per gram basis, kidney, liver, and lung were the major organs showing significant cumulative sIL-4R tissue levels (Table II). However, on an actual organ weight basis, the highest cumulative sIL-4R levels occurred in the blood, with liver being the major site of elimination. Of the sIL-4R observed in the blood, 43% was distributed to the liver.

V. SOLUBLE TNF RECEPTORS

A. Blood Clearance Comparisons

The clearance of intravenously administered sTNF-R monomer forms was compared to a sTNF-R fusion protein in mice. Although all blood clearance patterns could be described by two exponentials ($T_{1/2\alpha}$ and $T_{1/2\beta}$), major differences in clearance patterns and half-lives of these molecules were observed. The sTNF-R monomer expressed and purified from *E. coli* was cleared with a $T_{1/2\alpha}$ of 3.5 min and a $T_{1/2\beta}$ of 2.6 hr (Table IV). Of the injected sTNF-R (*E. coli*) dose, 93% was cleared during the distribution phase in 18 min with only the remaining 7% of the injected dose cleared in the second elimination phase. This rapid initial clearance was most likely kidney mediated as the $C_{\max}$ for the kidney occurred at 5 min and was fourfold greater than the blood $C_{\max}$. In addition, rapid kidney elimination was apparent, as the kidney $T_{1/2\beta}$ was 0.2 hr. The sTNF-R monomer expressed and purified from CHO cells was cleared with a $T_{1/2\alpha}$ of 11.6 min and a $T_{1/2\beta}$ of 3.8 hr. In this case, 62% of the injected TNF-R (CHO) dose was cleared during the initial phase in 58 min, with the remaining 38% cleared in the second phase in 19 hr. Clearance appeared kidney mediated, as the kidney $T_{1/2\beta}$ was 0.7 hr; however, the $C_{\max}$ for kidney was only 1.4-fold greater than the blood $C_{\max}$.

The sTNF-R fusion protein expressed and purified from BHK cells was

Table IV. Pharmacokinetic Parameters for TNF Receptors

	Type of sTNF-R administered[a]		
Parameters	Monomer (CHO)	Monomer (*E. coli*)	Fusion protein (BHK)
Blood kinetics			
C_{max}	47% ID/g	47% ID/g	62% ID/g
T_{max}	1 min	1 min	1 min
$T_{1/2\alpha}$	11.6 ± 2.3 min	3.5 ± 0.1 min	5.8 ± 2.4 min
$T_{1/2\beta}$	3.8 ± 0.8 hr	2.6 ± 0.3 hr	20.0 ± 3.9 hr
Tissue kinetics			
Kidney			
C_{max}	67% ID/g	203% ID/g	11% ID/g
T_{max}	5 min	5 min	1 min
$T_{1/2\beta}$	0.7 ± 0.2 hr	0.2 ± 0.01 hr	19.9 ± 2.6 hr
Liver			
C_{max}	12% ID/g	10% ID/g	26% ID/g
T_{max}	1 min	1 min	15 min
$T_{1/2\beta}$	3.3 ± 0.8 hr	3.5 ± 0.7 hr	13.9 ± 1.8 hr

[a] Mice were injected i.v. with TCA-precipitable, ^{125}I-labeled sTNF-R at the following dosages: 300 ng sTNF-R monomer (CHO), 444 ng sTNF-R monomer (*E. coli*), or 184 ng sTNF-R fusion protein (BHK). Data are presented as percentage of the injected dose (ID) per gram of tissue to allow direct comparisons among the parameters.

initially cleared with a $\tilde{T}_{1/2\alpha}$ of 5.8 min. Approximately 39% of the injected sTNF-R fusion protein was cleared during this phase in 26 min. The remaining 61% was cleared in a second elimination phase, with a $T_{1/2\beta}$ of 20 hr. Thus, the remaining injected sTNF-R fusion protein would be cleared in 100 hr or 4.2 days. Clearance of sTNF-R fusion protein appeared to be mainly liver mediated, as the liver $T_{1/2\beta}$ was 13.9 hr. A slow rate of liver clearance was apparent, as the liver C_{max} was less than half that of the blood C_{max} value.

B. Tissue Distribution of sTNF-R Monomer

For i.v. administration of sTNF-R monomer (CHO), cumulative tissue levels were observed mainly in blood, kidney, and lung on a per gram basis (Table II). However, when accounting for actual organ size or blood volume (8% body weight) on an organ (blood) weight basis, blood had the highest cumulative level. Lower levels were observed in both kidney and liver, with minimal levels observed in spleen, lung, and heart. Of the sTNF-R monomer (CHO) observed in blood, 37 and 24% distributed to kidneys and liver, respectively.

VI. COMPARISON OF sTNF-R FUSION PROTEIN TO sIL-4R FUSION PROTEIN

Blood Clearance Differences

The rationale for constructing fusion proteins is to facilitate ligand binding by constructing two monomeric receptors within one molecule and to prolong the half-life of the free monomeric receptor. Both sIL-4R and sTNF-R fusion proteins have been constructed and the blood kinetics compared to their respective monomeric forms (Fig. 1). As described above, less of the sTNF-R fusion protein was cleared in the initial distribution phase, with a greater percentage of the injected dose remaining in the circulation when compared to the sTNF-R monomer (CHO). The remaining 61% of the sTNF-R fusion protein was cleared slowly, with a $T_{1/2\beta}$ of 20 hr compared to the remaining 38% of the sTNF-R monomer (CHO) that was cleared with a $T_{1/2\beta}$ of 3.8 hr. In this instance, the fusion protein had a significantly prolonged half-life and thus greater bioavailability compared to the monomer. However, a similar pattern was not observed when the sIL-4R fusion protein was compared to the sIL-4R monomer. After a single bolus i.v. injection of sIL-4R fusion protein, 73% of the injected dose was cleared during the initial distribution phase with a $T_{1/2\alpha}$ of 2.5 ± 0.3 min, which was similar to 75% of the injected sIL-4R monomer cleared with a $T_{1/2}$ of 9 ± 1 min. For the sIL-4R fusion protein, the remaining 27% was cleared with a $T_{1/2\beta}$ of 2.9 ± 0.4 hr, which was comparable to the remaining 25% of the sIL-4R monomer cleared with a $T_{1/2\beta}$ of 2.3 ± 0.8 hr. Thus, there was no significant pharmacokinetic advantage of the sIL-4R fusion protein when compared to the monomeric receptor. Because the sIL-4R monomer rapidly accumulated in the liver, distribution of the sIL-4R fusion protein to the liver was investigated. Significantly greater and prolonged accumulation of the sIL-4R fusion protein was observed in the liver (Fig. 2). This greater accumulation most likely resulted in a more rapid clearance of sIL-4R fusion protein by the liver. Thus, the half-life for the sIL-4R fusion protein was comparable to the monomer instead of being prolonged, as would be expected for a larger fusion protein. In comparison, minimal levels of the sTNF-R fusion protein accumulated in the liver when compared to the sTNF-R monomer (Fig. 2). This minimal increase in the liver may have reflected the higher blood levels observed for the sTNF-R fusion protein.

VII. SUMMARY

The potential use of soluble cytokine receptors as therapeutics in disease states when excessive or prolonged cytokine expression leads to patho-

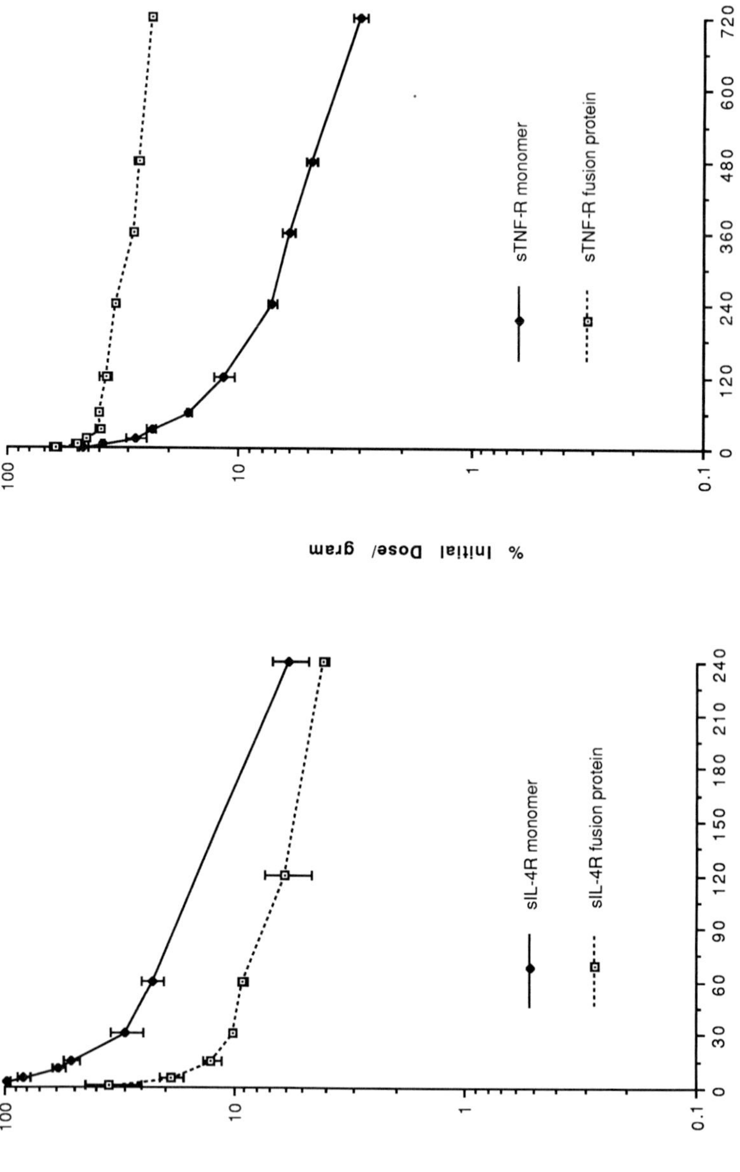

Fig. 1. Blood clearance of sIL-4R and sTNF-R comparing monomeric forms to fusion proteins. Mice were injected i.v. with TCA-precipitable, ^{125}I-radiolabeled soluble receptors in monomeric form or as dimeric fusion proteins. Mice were bled by cardiac puncture at various times. Data are presented as a percentage of the initial injected dose per gram of blood to allow direct comparisons. Each point represents the mean ± SEM (n = 3 mice).

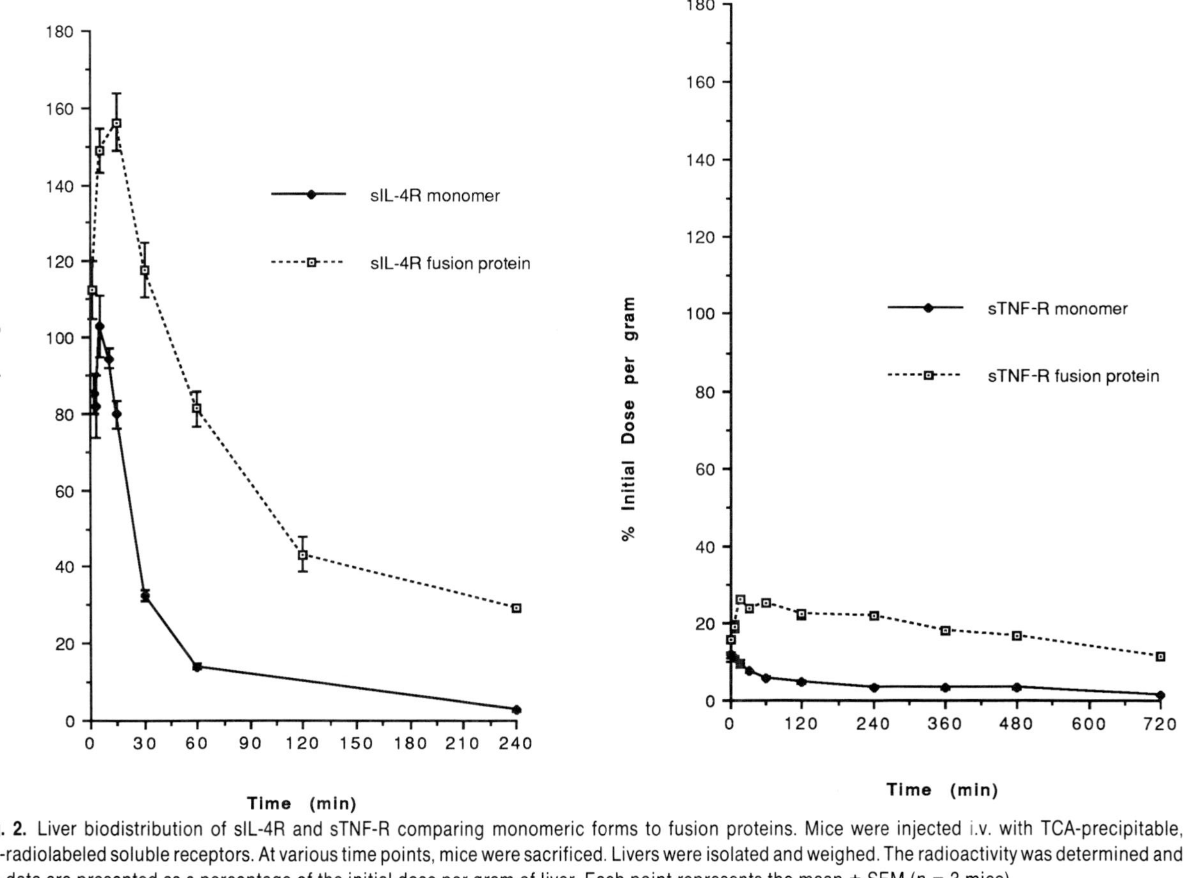

Fig. 2. Liver biodistribution of sIL-4R and sTNF-R comparing monomeric forms to fusion proteins. Mice were injected i.v. with TCA-precipitable, ^{125}I-radiolabeled soluble receptors. At various time points, mice were sacrificed. Livers were isolated and weighed. The radioactivity was determined and the data are presented as a percentage of the initial dose per gram of liver. Each point represents the mean ± SEM (n = 3 mice).

genesis is just beginning (Van Brunt, 1989). The inhibitory effects of soluble receptors have been found to be highly potent and specific for their respective cytokines (Maliszewski and Fanslow, 1990; Maliszewski *et al.,* 1990). Recent *in vivo* data have shown that exogenously administered soluble receptors can function as cytokine antagonists and suppress autoimmune inflammatory responses (Jacobs *et al.,* 1991a), allograft rejection, and alloreactivity (Fanslow *et al.,* 1990b). The proposed frequency of administration and dosage of a therapeutic agent is dependent on the half-life of the agent and the route of administration. The elimination or half-life of a drug usually depends on its physiochemical properties (molecular size, glycosylation, isoelectric point, and hydrophobic/hydrophilic properties) (DiPalma and DiGregorio, 1990; Katzung, 1984). The half-life will also depend on the mechanism of clearance for that specific receptor. Once pharmacokinetic data are available for soluble receptors, the therapeutic potential of these molecules can be better evaluated. Only limited pharmacokinetic data are currently available for soluble cytokine receptors (Jacobs *et al.,* 1991b).

For sIL-1R, the majority of an intravenously administered dose was cleared in the second elimination phase, with a reasonably long half-life (6.3 hr), such that the entire dose was not eliminated until 35 hr. If administration is by subcutaneous injection, the half-life was even more prolonged. One explanation for the prolonged half-life is the minimal distribution to liver and kidneys and thus low levels of clearance by these organs. In contrast, elimination of intravenously administered sIL-4R was relatively rapid, with a short half-life (2.3 hr). This appeared mainly due to liver distribution and clearance, which has been the highest observed for any soluble cytokine receptor. Administering sIL-4R by subcutaneous injection significantly prolonged the half-life. This was most likey due to delaying the rate of liver distribution by slowing the rate of sIL-4R absorption into the circulation. Thus, subcutaneous injection would be the recommended route of administration for this receptor. Construction of a larger dimeric sIL-4R fusion protein did not prolong the i.v. half-life compared to that of the monomer, as the sIL-4R fusion protein was distributed to, and was cleared by, the liver to a greater degree. Of the two sTNF-R monomers that were evaluated, the glycosylated monomer produced by CHO cells clearly had greater bioavailability, as less was cleared in the initial phase. In addition, the glycosylated monomer had a longer elimination half-life than did the unglycosylated monomer. For both sTNF-R monomers, clearance appeared to be mediated more by the kidneys than the liver. The dimeric sTNF-R fusion protein was cleared predominantly in the second phase and had a significantly prolonged half-life (20 hr) compared to the glycosylated monomeric form (3.8 hr). Clearance of the sTNF-R fusion protein appeared to be primarily liver mediated, but at a signficantly lower rate compared to the sIL-4R fusion protein. Thus, the difference in hepatic clearance most likely is the reason for the tremendous difference in pharmacokinetic patterns. Though construction of a fusion protein can provide an effective method of prolonging the serum half-life of a soluble cytokine receptor, it does not guarantee it.

In summary, pharmacokinetic parameters appear to vary for each receptor and for different forms of the same receptor. Thus, it will be important to analyze the pharmacokinetic parameters and biodistribution patterns for individual soluble receptors to predict their therapeutic potential and/or administration requirements for clinical trials.

Acknowledgments

The authors thank Eileen Roux, Robert Miller, Ky Clifford, Dauphine Torrance, Tim Sato, Tim VandenBos, and Denise Dupont for their excellent technical assistance; Jennifer Slack and Drs. Steve Dower and Craig Smith for their assistance in radiolabeling the receptors; and Kathy Sarkanen for preparation of the manuscript. All fusion proteins were constructed by Behringwerke.

References

DiPalma, J. R., and DiGregorio, G. J. (1990). *In* "Basic Pharmacology in Medicine," p. 31. McGraw-Hill, New York.

Dower, S. K., Wignall, J. M., Schooley, K., McMahan, C. J., Jackson, J. L., Prickett, K. S., Lupton, S., Cosman, D., and Sims, J. E. (1989). *J. Immunol.* **142**, 4314.

Fanslow, W. C., Clifford, K., VandenBos, T., Teel, A., Armitage, R. J., and Beckmann, M. P. (1990a). *Cytokine* **2**, 398.

Fanslow, W. C., Sims, J. E., Sassenfeld, H., Morrissey, P. J., Gillis, S., Dower, S. K., and Widmer, M. (1990b). *Science* **248**, 739–742.

Fernandez-Botran, R. (1991). *FASEB J.* **5**, 2567–2574.

Gennuso, R., Spigelman, M. K., Vallabhajosula, S., Moore, F., Zappulla, R. A., Nieves, J., Strauchen, J. A., Paciucci, P. A., Malis, L. I., Goldsmith, S. J., and Holland, J. F. (1989). *J. Biol. Response Modif.* **8**, 375.

Gustavson, L. E., Nadeau, R. W., and Oldfield, N. F. (1989). *J. Biol. Response Modif.* **8**, 440.

Jacobs, C. A., Baker, P. E., Roux, E. R., Picha, K. S., Toivola, B., Waugh, S., and Kennedy, M. K. (1991a). *J. Immunol.* **146**, 2983–2989.

Jacobs, C., Lynch, D. H., Roux, E. R., Miller, R., Davis, B., Widmer, M. B., Wignall, J., VandenBos, T., Park, L. S., and Beckmann, M. P. (1991b). *Blood* **77**, 2396–2403.

Katzung, B. G. (1984). *In* "Basic and Clinical Pharmacology," p. 23. Lange Med. Publ., Los Altos, California.

Maliszewski, C. R., and Fanslow, W. C. (1990). *TibTech* **8**, 324–329.

Maliszewski, C. R., Sato, T. A., VandenBos, T., Waugh, S., Dower, S. K., Slack, J., Beckmann, M. P., and Grabstein, K. H. (1990). *J. Immunol.* **144**, 3028–3033.

Paul, W. E. (1989). *Cell* **57**, 521–524.

Smith, K. A. (1990). *Eur. Cytokine Network* **1**, 7–13.

Van Brunt, J. (1989). *Bio/Technology* **7**, 668–669.

Immunomodulation with Soluble IFN-γ Receptor: Preliminary Study

Laurence Ozmen, Michael Fountoulakis, Reiner Gentz, and Gianni Garotta
Pharmaceutical Research, New Technologies
Hoffmann-La Roche Ltd.
CH-4002 Basel, Switzerland

I. INTRODUCTION

Interferon-γ (IFN-γ) is distinct from IFN-α and IFN-β on account of its biological properties, i.e., inducing stimuli, types of cells producing it, sensitivity to acidic pH, and antigenic characteristics. IFN-γ, a product of NK cells and of activated T lymphocytes, was first characterized by its antiviral and antiproliferative activities (Trinchieri and Perussia, 1985; Vilcek *et al.,* 1985). However, most of the studies indicate that IFN-γ is an immunomodulatory and proinflammatory lymphokine (Table I). It promotes functional maturation of both T and B lymphocytes and modulates the early phases of antigen recognition through the regulation of expression of class I and II histocompatibility antigens. In the case of T lymphocytes, differentiation of both cytotoxic and helper cells appears to require both IFN-γ and interleukin-2 (IL-2). The proliferation and differentiation of B lymphocytes

Table I. Immunomodulatory and Proinflammatory Effects of IFN-γ

Cell	Effect
T cells	Promotes maturation and proliferation; induces MHC class I antigens, adhesion molecules; inhibits IL-4 synthesis
B cells	Promotes Ig synthesis, switch to IgG_{2a}; induces MHC class I antigens; inhibits IgE synthesis
Macrophages	Promotes adhesion; induces MHC class I and II antigens, Fc and adhesion molecule receptors, plasminogen-activator receptor, IL-1, TNF, chemotactic factors, release of proteolytic enzymes, O_2^-; NO_2, killing of microbes and tumor cells
PMNs	Promotes release of enzymes and radicals
Endothelial cells	Induces MHC class I and II antigens, adhesion molecules, IL-6, chemotactic factors
Epithelial cells	Induces MHC class I and II antigens, adhesion molecules
Fibroblasts	Induces fibronectin synthesis; inhibits collagen synthesis, proliferative effect of PDGF

are regulated by several interleukins, among which IFN-γ acts as cell growth-promoting factor, enhances the production of IgG_{2a}, and inhibits other IgG subclasses or IgE. On macrophages, IFN-γ induces the synthesis of both IL-1 and TNF, regulates the secretion of enzymes and cytotoxic molecules, and induces the expression of receptors for chemoattractants and plasminogen activator. Moreover, IFN-γ makes the normal endothelial cells become pro-coagulant, permeable, and markedly adhesive for granulocytes and mono-cytes (for review see Landolfo and Garotta, 1991).

Several animal experiments confirm the immunomodulatory and proin-flammatory activity of IFN-γ. It has been postulated that the induction of class II antigens in cells that are normally negative for it enables these cells to present their own structures as autoantigens and results in autoimmunity, e.g., type I diabetes or lupus erythematosus.

Thus, inhibitors of IFN-γ activity may be therapeutic agents for the sup-pression of alloreactions and the control of autoimmune disorders or chronic inflammations. Because IFN-γ exerts its biological activity through a single type of ubiquitous cell receptor (IFN-γR); the soluble form of such a receptor may be a tool to identify IFN-γ antagonists. Because of the species-specific interaction between IFN-γ and its receptor, soluble forms of both human and mouse IFN-γR were constructed. The human soluble IFN-γR was used *in vitro* for the screening of human IFN-γ (HuIFN-γ) antagonists, whereas the mouse soluble IFN-γR was used *in vivo* as a prototype of the IFN-γ antagonist.

II. IFN-γ RECEPTOR

The receptors for human and mouse IFN-γ (Aguet *et al.,* 1988; Cofano *et al.,* 1990; Gray *et al.,* 1989; Hemmi *et al.,* 1989; Kumar *et al.,* 1989; Munro and

Maniatis, 1989) have been recently cloned. The gene for human IFN-γR is located on the long arm of chromosome 6 (Rashidbaigi *et al.*, 1986); the gene for mouse IFN-γR is on mouse chromosome 10 (Mariano *et al.*, 1987). The human gene encodes a mature protein of 472 amino acids and a signal peptide of 17 residues. Hydropathy index computation of the translated sequence reveals a hydrophobic domain in the middle of the molecule (amino acids 230–249), compatible with a transmembrane-anchoring portion. The extracellular domain of the IFN-γR protein (amino acids 1–229) includes eight cysteines and five putative N-glycosylation sites; four cysteines and two putative N-glycosylation sites are present in the cytosolic domain of the receptor (amino acids 250–472) (Garotta *et al.*, 1990). The mature mouse IFN-γR protein is 451 amino acids long and contains a hydrophobic domain in the middle of the molecule, located between amino acids 228 and 252. IFN-γ is species specific and binds only the species-specific receptor. The sequences of human and mouse IFN-γR proteins show 54% homology (Munro and Maniatis, 1989), whereas the homology between human and mouse IFN-γ proteins is 40%. Eight out of the 10 cysteine residues of the extracellular domain and one out of two cysteine residues of the intracellular domain of the mouse receptor are conserved in the human protein (Kumar *et al.*, 1989).

III. SOLUBLE IFN-γR

As shown by epitope mapping with monoclonal antibodies (Garotta *et al.*, 1990) and by partial proteolysis (Fountoulakis *et al.*, 1991a), almost the full extracellular domain contributes to the binding site of HuIFN-γR. Accordingly, cDNAs encoding the extracellular domain of human and mouse IFN-γR were engineered and expressed as soluble receptors in *Spodoptera frugiperda* insect cells infected with recombinant baculoviruses (Gentz *et al.*, 1992). Because these cells can process proteins as higher eukaryotes do, they cleave off the signal peptide and the soluble IFN-γR starts as the mature proteins and terminates with the last amino acid of the extracellular domain (Ser at position 229 for HuIFN-γR, Ser at position 227 for MoIFN-γR) (Fig. 1). These proteins are secreted into the culture medium at 5–15 mg/liter and both human and mouse soluble IFNγ-R were purified through four chromatography steps: (1) Matrex blue, which separated certain hydrophobic proteins; (2) concanavalin A–Sepharose, which bound proteins carrying glucose and mannose sugar moieties, (3) polybuffer exchanger, which separated most of the other glycoproteins from the soluble receptor, and (4) Sephadex G-100, which removed all the remaining impurities and delivered a pure, soluble IFNγ-R with an overall recovery of 30% (Fountoulakis *et al.*, 1991b). The soluble receptors are stable proteins that retain full binding capacity after 30 days at 4°C or at room temperature.

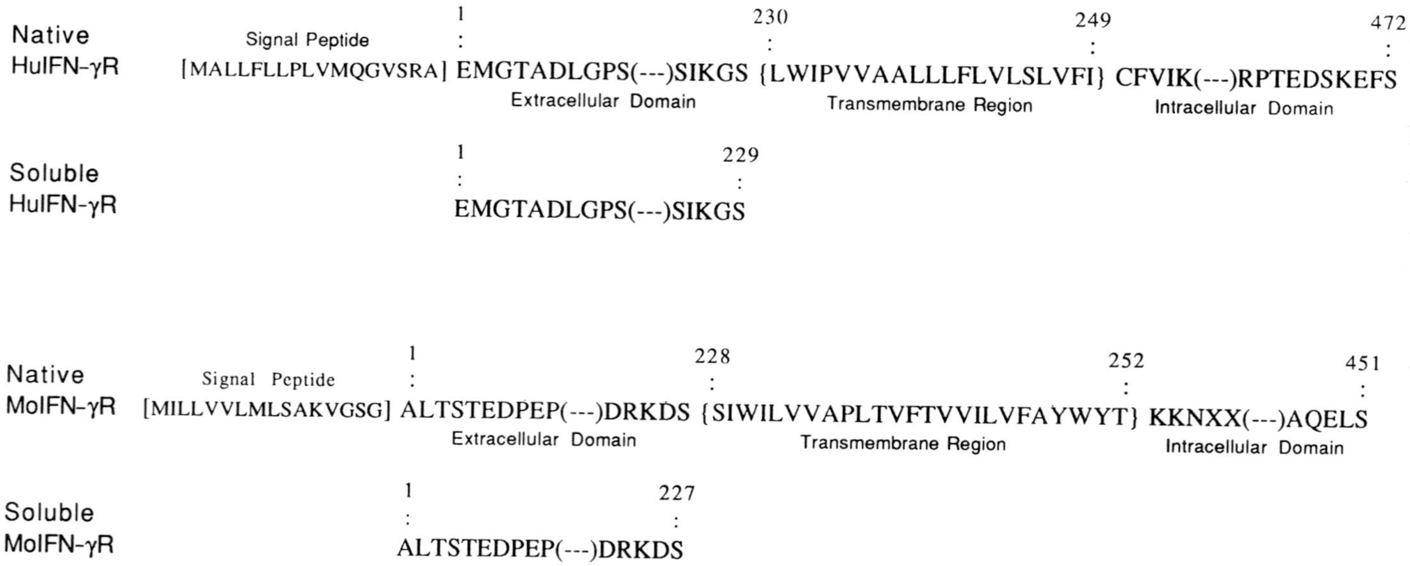

Native
HuIFN–γR

Signal Peptide 1 230 249 472
[MALLFLLPLVMQGVSRA] EMGTADLGPS(---)SIKGS {LWIPVVAALLLFLVLSLVFI} CFVIK(---)RPTEDSKEFS

Extracellular Domain Transmembrane Region Intracellular Domain

Soluble
HuIFN-γR

1 229
EMGTADLGPS(---)SIKGS

Native
MoIFN–γR

Signal Peptide 1 228 252 451
[MILLVVLMLSAKVGSG] ALTSTEDPEP(---)DRKDS {SIWILVVAPLTVFTVVILVFAYWYT} KKNXX(---)AQELS

Extracellular Domain Transmembrane Region Intracellular Domain

Soluble
MoIFN-γR

1 227
ALTSTEDPEP(---)DRKDS

Fig. 1. Construction of human and mouse soluble IFN-γ receptors.

Table II. Characterization of the Human and Mouse Soluble IFN-γ Receptors

Protein	Molecular mass (kDa)	Glycosylation (%)	IFN-γ AVA[a] (IC50, μg/ml)	Affinity (K_i, nM)
HuIFN-γR	30–32	25	1.5	0.55
MoIFN-γR	32–34	25	0.3	0.15

[a] AVA, Antiviral activity.

The soluble receptors were checked *in vitro* for their capacity to compete with the native receptor for the binding of radiolabed IFN-γ and to neutralize IFN-γ-mediated antiviral activity (AVA). The HuIFN-γR inhibits the binding of radiolabeled HuIFN-γ to the native receptor of human Raji cells (K_i = 0.5 nM) and neutralizes the antiviral activity that HuIFN-γ exerted on WISH cells infected with encephalomyocarditis virus (EMCV). In the same way, MoIFN-γR competes for the binding of radiolabeled MoIFN-γ to the native receptor of L1210 cells (K_i = 0.1 nM) and neutralizes the antiviral activity that MoIFN-γ exerted on L929 mouse fibroblasts (Table II).

IV. IMMUNOGENICITY AND PHARMACOKINETIC STUDIES OF MOUSE SOLUBLE IFN-γR

Soluble MoIFN-γR was used to study the possible therapeutic applications of an IFN-γ antagonist in mouse models of human diseases. The pharmacokinetics and the immunogenicity were first evaluated. On the basis of these studies and of the *in vitro* characterization of the MoIFN-γR activity, a schedule for the treatment of animals was planned.

A. Immunogenicity

The immunogenicity was assessed following two protocols. The first protocol consisted of four injections of 10 μg of MoIFN-γR emulsified in Freund's adjuvant every 2 weeks. No specific antibodies were detected in the sera of mice injected with MoIFN-γR, whereas animals receiving HuIFN-γR developed high titers of specific antibodies. The second protocol consisted of biweekly injections of soluble receptor for 2 months. This approach mimics a therapeutic use of the mouse receptor in mice. After 2 weeks, only the control mice injected with 1 or 10 μg of soluble HuIFN-γR developed specific antibodies (titers of 3000–40,000). After 2 months, 60% of the mice injected with 10 μg of soluble MoIFN-γR produced antibodies (maximal titer, 2000) that reacted with the receptor protein in an enzyme-linked immunoassay (ELISA) but did not recognize it in a Western blot (Table III).

Table III. Antigenicity of HuIFN-γR and MoIFN-γR after Chronic Injections in Mice[a]

Injection no.	HuIFN-γR (1 μg)	MoIFN-γR (100 μg)
0	0%	0%
3	0%	
4		0%
5	80%	
9	100%	
10		0%
13	100%	40%
16	100%	
19		60%

[a] Results are expressed as the percentage of positive mice (antibody titer >1000) in groups of five animals each.

B. Pharmacokinetics

In order to determine the optimal treatment schedule, mice were injected with 3 μg of iodinated soluble receptor. The presence of MoIFN-γR was evaluated by following the radioactivity in different tissues and in the sera of the treated animals. After i.p. injection, the half-life of the soluble MoIFN-γR was estimated to be 6 hr in the lymphoid organs and 3 hr in the sera. To confirm such an evaluation and to make sure that the radioactivity in the blood remained associated to fully active MoIFN-γR protein, the concentration of active MoIFN-γR present in standard solutions or animal sera was measured by the ability of these samples to inhibit the binding of radio-labeled MoIFN-γR to affinity-purified rabbit anti-MoIFN-γR antibodies. In this experiment, mice were injected with 100 μg of MoIFN-γR. Titration of the protein in the animal sera gave a blood half-life of only 1 hr. According to these results and taking into account the ability of MoIFN-γR to neutralize *in vitro* the antiviral activity that MoIFN-γ exerted on L929 mouse fibroblasts, the administration of 100 μg per mouse every second day should maintain an effective blood concentration.

V. MODULATION OF GRAFT-VERSUS-HOST DISEASE BY SOLUBLE MoIFN-γR

A. Modulation of Acute GVHD

Acute graft-versus-host disease (GVHD) was induced in (C57Bl/6 $\times$ DBA/2)F$_1$ (BDF$_1$) mice by injecting C57Bl/6 lymphoid cells. This reaction requires both donor Lyt-1$^+$ and Lyt-2$^+$ cells and is characterized by severe hypoplasia, aplastic anemia, and hypogammaglobulinemia (Gleichmann *et al.,* 1984). Allogeneic host cells activate the donor Lyt-1$^+$ lymphocytes, which then provide maximal help to donor Lyt-2$^+$ suppressive lymphocytes (Rolink and Gleichmann, 1983).

Starting from day 0, when the allogeneic cells were injected, the animals were given 100 μg of MoIFN-γR every second day for 2 months. The treatment with MoIFN-γR prevented weight loss, reduced mortality (31 vs. 61%), and inhibited the rise of serum amyloid protein (SAP) (Table IV). The level of this acute-phase reactant correlates with the severity of the GVHD (Bayston *et al.,* 1990). Smith and co-workers (1991) showed that the suppressive activity found in the spleen of mice suffering from GVHD could be reverted *in vitro* by antibodies that neutralize the activity of IFN-γ. Alloreactive donor Lyt-1$^+$ cells were detected in the spleens of long-term GVHD F_1 chimeras; alloreactive Lyt-2$^+$ cells were no longer found (Pals *et al.,* 1984). This Lyt-1$^+$ population of the GVHD spleen seems to be the source of the high levels of IFN-γ. The mortality rate likely did not increase when the treatment with MoIFN-γR was discontinued because the Lyt-1$^+$ population played a crucial role in the early phase of GVHD.

B. Modulation of Chronic GVHD

BDF_1 mice injected with DBA/2 parental cells develop a chronic GVHD. It is triggered by the donor Lyt-1$^+$ cells, which are activated by the allogeneic MHC class II structures of the host B cells (Gleichmann *et al.,* 1984), and it is characterized by persistent lymphoid hyperplasia, hypergammaglob-

Table IV. MoIFN-γR in Acute GVHD: Injection of C57Bl/6 Cells in BDF_1 Mice

Months postinjection	Splenocytes injected	MoIFN-γR treatment[a]	Body weight[b]	SAP[c]
0	BDF_1	−	26 (1)	3.5 (2)
0	BDF_1	+	28 (1)	5 (4)
0	C57Bl/6	−	27 (2)	9 (7)
0	C57Bl/6	+	28 (2)	15 (11)
2	BDF_1	−	32 (1)	5 (1)
2	BDF_1	+	34 (1)	5 (1)
2	C57Bl/6	−	28 (7)	51 (101)
2	C57Bl/6	+	35 (2)	8 (8)

[a] 100 μg of MoIFN-γR in saline was injected i.p. 3 times a week for 2 months.
[b] Values in grams; SD in parentheses.
[c] SAP, Serum amyloid protein. Values in μg/ml; SD in parentheses.

Table V. MoIFN-γR in Chronic GVHD: Injection of DBA/2 Cells in BDF₁ Mice

| | | | Mortality rate[b] | |
| | | | Months after cell injection | |
Autoantibody	Splenocytes injected	MoIFN-γR treatment[a]	0	2
Anti-dsDNA	BDF₁	−	0/5	0/5
Anti-dsDNA	BDF₁	+	0/4	0/4
Anti-dsDNA	DBA/2	−	0/12	7/12
Anti-dsDNA	DBA/2	+	1/11	1/11

[a] 100 μg of MoIFN-γR in saline was injected i.p. 3 times a week for 2 months.
[b] Number of mice that died/number of mice treated.

ulinemia, autoantibodies characteristic of systemic lupus erythematousus (SLE), immunoglobulin deposition in the skin, and severe immune complex glomerulonephritis (ICGN) (Gleichmann *et al.,* 1982; Van Rappard van der Veen *et al.,* 1983). The generation of autoantibodies by the host B cells is induced by donor T helper cells that recognize class II-restricted autoantigens on the surface of host B cells (Morris *et al.,* 1990). Treatment with 100 μg of MoIFN-γR every second day significantly reduced the serum level of anti-DNA autoantibodies (especially of the IgG_{2a} isotype) without affecting the mortality rate (Table V). The anti-DNA autoantibodies increased to the placebo level after the treatment was discontinued. This mouse SLE-like disease and human SLE show the same types of autoantibodies (Gleichmann *et al.,* 1982; Portanova *et al.,* 1985; Van Rappard van der Veen *et al.,* 1984). However, the typical exacerbation and remission phases of human SLE are not observed. During the exacerbation phases (rash, oral ulcers, alopecia, arthralgia), higher anti-DNA levels are detected in the patients' sera (Isenberg *et al.,* 1984). A similar incidence of ICGN-induced mortality observed in treated and nontreated animals suggests the need for a long-lasting MoIFN-γR treatment.

VI. DISCUSSION

Several animal experiments demonstrate the disease-promoting activity of IFN-γ in autoimmunity and alloreactions and suggest the need for testing the potential therapeutic activity of soluble MoIFN-γR in chronic GVHD, which is an induced model of SLE, and in acute GVHD, which is a model of alloreaction.

It has been postulated that the induction of class II antigens in cells that are normally negative for them enable these cells to present their own structures as autoantigens, resulting in autoimmunity, i.e., type I diabetes, thyroiditis, encephalomyelitis, and lupus erythematosus. It is particularly striking to find that patients with thyroiditis or type I diabetes strongly express MHC class II antigens in thyrocytes (Todd *et al.,* 1987) or islet β cells. Nicoletti and co-workers (1990) showed that treatment with monoclonal antibodies that neutralize the activity of rat IFN-γ prevents diabetes onset in BB/wor rats. Systemic injections of the β cell toxin streptozotocin in susceptible mice result in a form of diabetes resembling human insulin-dependent type I diabetes. The onset of disease is retarded by immunosuppressive agents and exacerbated by IFN-γ (Campbell *et al.,* 1988). Moreover, the transgenic mice expressing the gene for IFN-γ under the control of the insulin promoter spontaneously developed type I diabetes (Sarvetnick *et al.,* 1990).

F_1 hybrids between autoimmune NZB mice and phenotypically normal NZW mice develop severe systemic autoimmune disease with a fatal immune complex glumerulonephritis similar to human systemic lupus erythematosus. Treatment with IFN-γ accelerated the development of nephritis, whereas antibodies to IFN-γ blocked or delayed the progression of the disease (Jacob *et al.,* 1987).

Using monoclonal antibodies to murine IFN-γ in a limiting dilution assay, it was shown that the neutralization of this lymphokine inhibits the IL-2-dependent growth and maturation of single cytolytic T lymphocyte (CTL) precursors (Farrar *et al.,* 1981; Simon *et al.,* 1979). Recently, Maraskovsky and co-workers (1989) showed that both IL-2 and IFN-γ are required for the majority of CTL precursors to develop into CTL clones. Parallel *in vivo* experiments showed that a mAb neutralizing IFN-γ impairs the development of alloreative CTLs, and the rejection of tumor, skin, or heart allografts is suppressed or delayed when the recipients are treated with antibodies neutralizing IFN-γ (Landolfo *et al.,* 1985; Didlake *et al.,* 1988).

The soluble receptors of cytokines may represent a natural feedback mechanism to prevent overstimulation. There is evidence of natural occurrence of soluble receptors for GH, EGF, NGF, TNF, IL-1, IL-2, IL-4, IL-7, and IFN-γ. The function of these natural forms of soluble receptors has not yet been elucidated. The production of soluble receptors for IL-4, IL-7, or EGF may be due to an alternative splicing of the surface receptor-encoding gene (Goodwin *et al.,* 1990; Mosley *et al.,* 1989; Weber *et al.,* 1984), whereas TNF, IL-2, and most likely IL-1 soluble receptors derive from the proteolytic cleavage of the cellularly expressed receptor (Gatanaga *et al.,* 1990; Giri *et al.,* 1990; Nophar *et al.,* 1990; Robb and Kutny, 1987). Novick and co-workers (1989) described the presence of natural IFN-γ soluble receptors and IL-6 soluble receptors in normal human urine. The finding of the IFN-γ soluble receptor in urine has not yet been confirmed in other body fluids under normal or pathological situations, but the presence of such a receptor in human urine could be explained by the shedding of the cellular receptor, which is highly expressed on kidney tubular cells (Valente *et al.,* 1992).

The use of recombinant soluble IFN-γR *in vivo* confirmed the role of IFN-γ in some pathologies and demonstrated the potential IFN-γ antagonistic activity of such a molecule. Because of their short half-lives and their administration route, soluble receptors do not represent the ideal therapeutic agent; nevertheless, they may be useful tools to study the possible applications of cytokine antagonists in pathological situations.

VII. SUMMARY

Several *in vivo* experiments support the hypothesis that an IFN-γ antagonist may have therapeutic applications in autoimmune diseases, hypersensitivities, and alloreactions. IFN-γ exerts its biological activity through the binding to a single-chain cell surface receptor. The protein that corresponds to the external domain of mouse IFN-γ receptor was expressed in insect cells infected with recombinant baculovirus; this protein was characterized and used *in vivo* as a prototype of the IFN-γ antagonist. This protein does not show any strong antigenicity after *in vivo* injection in mice. Despite a blood half-life of only 1–3 hr as demonstrated in pharmacokinetic experiments, the mouse soluble IFN-γR was able to modify the onset of acute GVHD (alloreaction) and chronic GVHD (lupuslike disease).

References

Aguet, M., Dembic, Z., and Merlin, G. (1988). *Cell* **55**, 273.

Bayston, K. F., Huby, R., and Cohen, J. (1990). *Clin. Exp. Immunol.* **81**, 239.

Campbell, I. L., Oxbrow, L., Koulmanda, M., and Harrison, L. C. (1988). *J. Immunol.* **140**, 1111.

Cofano, F., Moore, S. F., Tanaka, S., Yuhki, N., Landolfo, S., and Appella, E. (1990). *J. Biol. Chem.* **265**, 4064.

Didlake, R. H., Kim, E. K., Sheehan, K., Schreiber, R. D., and Kahan, B. D. (1988). *Transplantation* **45**, 222.

Farrar, W. L., Johnson, H. M., and Farrar, J. J. (1981). *J. Immunol.* **126**, 1120.

Fountoulakis, M., Lahm, H. W., Maris, A., Friedlein, A., Manneberg, M., Stüber, D., and Garotta, G. (1991a). *J. Biol. Chem.* **266**, 14970.

Fountoulakis, M., Schlaeger, E. J., Gentz, R., Juranville, J. F., Manneberg, M., Ozmen, L., and Garotta, G. (1991b). *Eur. J. Biochem.* **198**, 441.

Garotta, G., Ozmen, L., Fountoulakis, M., Dembic, Z., van Loon, A. P. G. M., and Stüber, D. (1990). *J. Biol. Chem.* **265**, 6908.

Gatanaga, T., Hwang, C., Kohr, W., Cappuccini, F., Lucci, J. A., Jeffes, E. W. B., Lentz, R., Tomich, J., Yamamoto, R. S., and Granger, G. A. (1990). *Proc. Natl. Acad. Sci. U.S.A.* **87**, 8781.

Gentz, R., Hayes, A., Grau, N., Fountoulakis, M., Lahm, H. W., Ozmen, L., and Garotta, G. (1992). *Eur. J. Biochem.* (in press).

Giri, J. G., Newton, R. C., and Horuk, R. (1990). *J. Biol. Chem.* **265**, 17146.

Gleichmann, E., Van Elven, E. H., and Van der Veen, J. P. W. (1982). *Eur. J. Immunol.* **12,** 152.

Gleichmann, E., Pals, S. T., Rolink, A. G., Radaszkiewicz, T., and Gleichmann, H. (1984). *Immunol. Today* **5,** 324.

Goodwin, R. G., Friend, D., Ziegler, S. F., Jerzy, R., Falk, B. A., Gimpel, S., Cosman, D., Dower, S. K., March, C. J., Namen, A. E., and Park, L. S. (1990). *Cell* **60,** 941.

Gray, P. W., Leong, S., Fennie, E. H., Farrar, M. A., Pingel, J. T., Fernandez-Luna, J., and Schreiber, R. D. (1989). *Proc. Natl. Acad. Sci. U.S.A.* **86,** 8497.

Hemmi, S., Peghini, P., Metzler, M., Merlin, G., Dembic, Z., and Aguet, M. (1989). *Proc. Natl. Acad. Sci. U.S.A.* **86,** 9901.

Isenberg, D. A., Schoenfeld, Y., and Madaio, M. (1984). *Lancet* **ii,** 417.

Jacob, C. O., van der Meide, P. H., and McDevitt, M. O. (1987). *J. Exp. Med.* **166,** 798.

Kumar, C. S., Muthukumaran, G., Frost, L. J., Noe, M., Ahn, Y. H., Mariano, T. M., and Pestka, S. (1989). *J. Biol. Chem.* **264,** 17939.

Landolfo, S., and Garotta, G. (1991). *J. Immunol Res* **9,** 81.

Landolfo, S., Cofano, F., Giovarelli, M., Prat, M., Cavallo, G., and Forni, G. (1985). *Science* **229,** 176.

Maraskovsky, E., Chen, W. F., and Shortman, K. (1989). *J. Immunol.* **143,** 1210.

Mariano, T. M., Kozak, C. A., Langer, J. A., and Pestka, S. (1987). *J. Biol. Chem.* **262,** 5812.

Morris, S. C., Cheek, R. L., Cohen, P. L., and Eisenberg, R. A. (1990). *J. Exp. Med.* **171,** 503.

Mosley, B., Beckmann, P., March, C. J., Idzerda, R. L., Gimpel, S. D., Vanden Bos, T., Friend, D., Alpert, A., Anderson, D., Jackson, J., Wignall, J. M., Smith, C., Gallis, B., Sims, J. E., Urdal, D., Widmer, M. B., Cosman, D., and Park, L. S. (1989). *Cell* **59,** 335.

Munro, S., and Maniatis, T. (1989). *Proc. Natl. Acad. Sci. U.S.A.* **86,** 9248.

Nicoletti, F., Meroni, P. L., Landolfo, S., Gariglio, M., Guzzardi, S., Darcellini, W., Lunotta, M., Mughini, L., and Zanussi, C. (1990). *Lancet* No. 336, 319.

Nophar, Y., Kemper, O., Brakebusch, C., Engelmann, H., Zwang, R., Aderka, D., Holtmann, H., and Wallach, D. (1990). *EMBO J.* **9,** 3269.

Novick, D., Engelmann, H., Wallach, D., and Rubinstein, M. (1989). *J. Exp. Med.* **170,** 1409.

Pals, S. T., Gleichmann, H., and Gleichmann, E. (1984). *J. Exp. Med.* **159,** 508.

Portanova, J. P., Claman, H. N., and Kotzin, B. L. (1985). *J. Immunol.* **135,** 3850.

Rashidbaigi, A., Lancer, J. A., Jung, V., Jones, C., and Morse, H. G. (1986). *Proc. Natl. Acad. Sci. U.S.A.* **83,** 384.

Robb, R. J., and Kutny, R. M. (1987). *J. Immunol.* **139,** 855.

Rolink, A. G., and Gleichmann, E. (1983). *J. Exp. Med.* **158,** 546.

Sarvetnick, N., Shizuru, J., Liggitt, D., Martin, L., McIntyre, B., Gregory, A., Parslow, T., and Stewart, T. (1990). *Nature (London)* **346,** 844.

Simon, P. L., Farrar, J. J., and King, P. D. (1979). *J. Immunol.* **127,** 1222.

Smith, S. R., Terminelli, C., Kernworthy-Bott, L., and Phillips, D. L. (1991). *Cell. Immunol.* **134,** 336.

Trinchieri, G., and Perussia, B. (1985). *Immunol. Today* **6,** 131.

Todd, I., Pujol-Borrell, R., Hammond, L. J., McNally, J. M., Feldmann, M., and Bottazzo, G. F. (1987). *Clin. Exp. Immunol.* **69,** 524.

Valente, G., Ozmen, L., Novelli, F., Palestro, G., Forni, G., and Garotta, G. (1992). *Eur. J. Immunol.* **22,** 2403.

Van Rappard van der Veen, F. M., Radaszkiewicz, T., Terraneo, L., and Gleichmann, E. (1983). *J. Immunol.* **130,** 2693

Van Rappard van der Veen, F. M., Kiesel, U., Schuler, W., Melief, C. J. M., Landegent, J., and Gleichmann, E. (1984). *J. Immunol.* **132,** 1814.

Vilcek, J., Gray, P. W., Rinderknecht, E., and Sevastopoulos, C. G. (1985). *Lymphokines* **11,** 1.

Weber, W., Gill, G. N., and Spiess, J. (1984). *Science* **224,** 294.

TNF Receptor Distribution in Human Tissues

Bernhard Ryffel
Institut für Toxikologie
Eidgenössischen Technischen Hochschule
Universität Zürich
CH-8603 Schwerzenbach/Zürich, Switzerland

M. J. Mihatsch
Institut für Pathologie
Universität Basel
CH-4003 Basel, Switzerland

I. INTRODUCTION

Tumor necrosis factor (TNF) plays an important role in host defenses against infection and in inflammation (1–3). The biological significance of TNF and its role in various diseases are still areas of intensive research. TNF consists of two homologous peptide factors (4), TNF-α, which is produced by activated monoytes, macrophages, and activated T lymphocytes (5,6), and TNF-β, which is derived from a subpopulation of activated T cells (7). TNF exerts its biological activity by binding to two types of cellular TNF receptors (8,9). Recent immunohistochemical investigations on the location of TNF-α production identified the germinal center dendritic reticulum cells (DRCs) as the main source of TNF-α in tissues (10,11). *In vitro* studies suggest a ubiquitous occurrence of TNF receptors (TNF-R), and TNF has been shown to exert important effects on lymphocytes (12–14), monocytes (15), fibroblasts, and on the endothelium (16,17).

International Review of Experimental Pathology, Volume 34B

In order to gain more insight into the immunoregulatory role of this locally produced cytokine, we investigated the nature of TNF-α-responsive cells *in situ* by examining the expression of the two TNF-R proteins *in situ* in lymphoid tissues. It was a reasonable assumption that the TNF-α-producing DRCs were unlikley to be the only cells responding to this cytokine. Both types of TNF-R have recently been characterized by molecular cloning and have been shown to differ in their apparent molecular weights (75,000 and 55,000) and in their relative expression on human cell lines (18–21). Monoclonal antibodies (mAbs) have been developed against the p75 TNF-R (utr series) and the p55 TNF-R (htr series) and were shown to be specific and non-cross-reactive (8), despite the high degree of sequence similarity in the extracellular region from both types of TNF-R (18).

Two mAbs suitable for immunohistochemistry, utr-1, a TNF-blocking anti-p75 antibody, and htr-19, a nonblocking anti-p55 TNF-R antibody, were used for this investigation.

II. DISTRIBUTION OF TNF-R IN LYMPHOID TISSUES

In the thymus, the immunoreactivity was mainly confined to the medulla (Fig. 1A). Medullary utr-1 (p75)-reactive cells comprised dendritic cells and lymphoblasts, which costained with the Tac protein of IL-2R (Fig. 1B). No utr-1 reactivity was found either in thymic epithelium or in cortical thymocytes. There was a faint staining of dendritic cells with the htr-19 antibody. Hasall's bodies gave no reaction with either antibody.

Human bone marrow cells expressed neither the p75 nor the p55 protein. On peripheral blood lymphocytes, a faint membrane staining was obtained with utr-1 but not with htr-19.

In the spleen, utr-1-reactive cells, comprising dendritic cells and lymphoblasts, were mainly located in the T cell area (periarterial lymphatic sheath); only a few utr-1-reactive cells were found in the mantle zone and follicles of the B cell area.

Serial cryostat sections of lymph nodes were incubated with urt-1, htr-19, Tac (CD25), or T cell mAb. Incubation with the utr-1 mAb resulted in strong staining of interdigitating reticulum cells (IDCs) and of activated T lymphocytes in the interfollicular T cell area (Fib. 1C). The distribution of utr-1-reactive cells overlapped that of cells expressing the Il-2 receptor (Tac) in the T cell area (Fig. 1D). Based on sequential incubation with utr-1a and Tac on serial sections, it is concluded that utr-1-reactive lymphocytes and a subpopulation of IDC coexpress the Tac protein. The htr-19 immunoreactivity was confined to follicular dendritic cells (DRC) in germinal centers and was not found at other sites (Fig. 1E). The staining pattern with

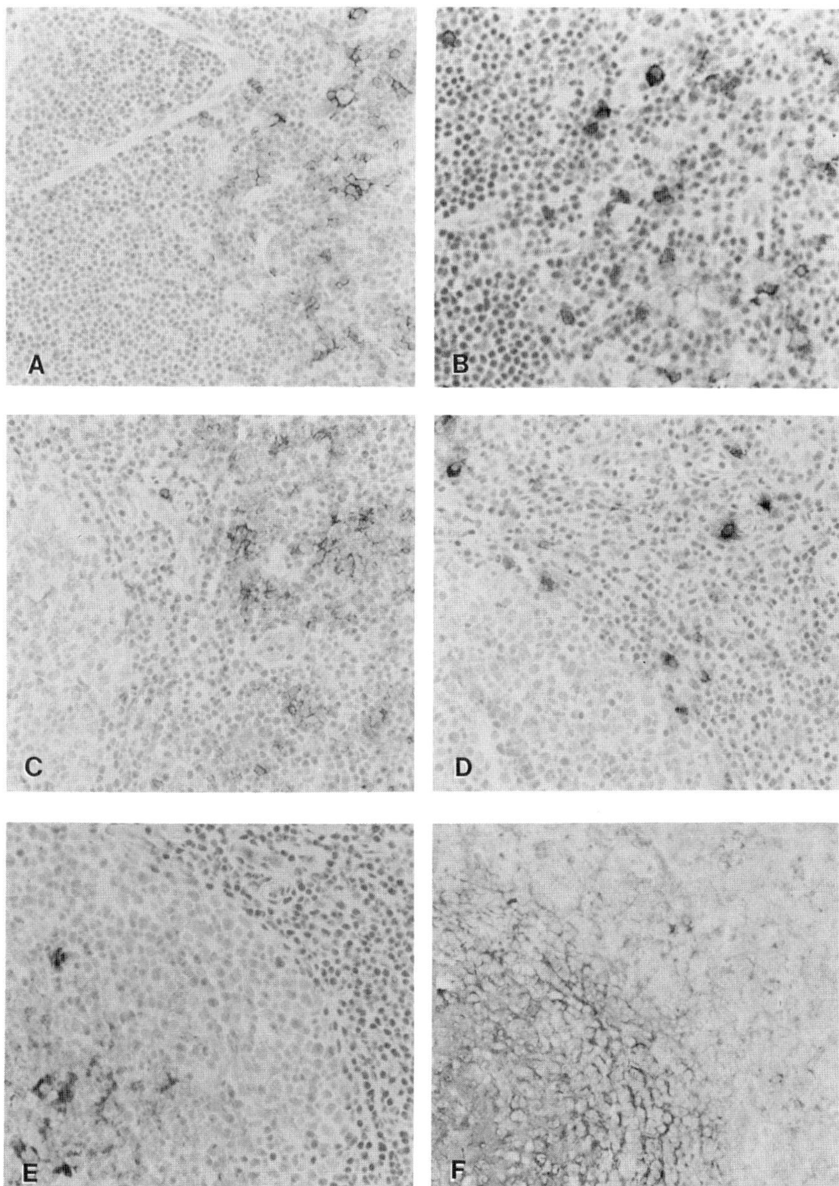

Fig. 1. Immunostaining for TNF receptor (A, C, D, and E), CD25 IL-2 receptor (B), and TNF-α (F) on cryostat sections of human thymus (A and B) and lymph node (C–F), using monoclonal antibodies and the APAAP technique ($\times$300). Thymus with utr-1-positive cells in the medulla (A) and CD25-positive cells at the same location (B). Lymph node with utr-1-reactive lymphocytes and IDCs in the interfollicular area (C) and CD25-positive cells in the same location (D); htr-19-reactive DRCs in the germinal center (E) and TNF-α immunostaining of germinal center cells, including DRCs.

htr-19 was comparable to that obtained with DRC1 antibody which stains specifically this cell population (not shown). The specificity of the immuno-reaction was supported by negative controls obtained by substitution or omission of the primary antibody, and by competition with excess TNF-α for utr-1 staining. In tonsils a staining pattern similar to that in lymph nodes was observed (Table I): few if any utr-1-reactive cells were found in germinal centers and the mantle zone of the follicle; the interfollicular T cell area (paracortex) gave distinct utr-1 staining of the DRCs and of T lymphocytes. Finally, the T6-positive Langerhans cells in the epithelium stained only with the urt-1 antibody. In the lymphoid tissues associated with the mucosae of the gut and the bronchus, a similar pattern of utr-1-reactive cells was found in the T cell areas.

Table I. Distribution of TNF-α Receptor Proteins in Normal Lymphoid Tissues

Organ[a]	n	Area[b]	TNF receptor protein utr-1	htr-19	IL2 receptor TAC	TNF-α
Tonsil	6	TA	+++	−	+++	+
		MZ	+	−	+	+
		GC	+	+	+	++
Lymph node	6	TA	+++	−	+++	(+)
		MZ	+	−	+	+
		GC	(+)	+	+	++
Spleen	3	TA	+++	−	++	−
		MZ	+	−	++	−
		GC	−	+	−	+
		RP	+	−	+	−
Thymus	2	Cortex	−	−	−	−
		Medulla	+++	+	++	−
Skin	2	Langerhans cells	++	−	+	−
Mucosa-associated lymphoid tissue	4	TA	+++	−	++	−
		MZ	+	−	+	−
		GC	(+)	+	(+)	+
Kidney	12	Reticulum cells (interstitial)	++	−	+	

[a] Organs examined that were negative included liver, heart, lungs, brain, adrenals, uterus, ovaries, testes, prostate, stomach, and intestines.

[b] Immunoreactivity within various areas (TA, T cell area; MZ, mantle zone or marginal zone for the spleen; GC, germinal center; RP, red pulp) was assessed by a semiquantitative score (0–3+).

III. TNF-R DISTRIBUTION IN OTHER TISSUES

The TNF-R distribution was also investigated in nonlymphoid tissue (Table I). Scattered utr-1-positive mononuclear cells in the interstitial space of the kidneys, the mucosae of various organs, and at inflammatory sites were observed. In inflammatory lesions, utr-1-reactive mononuclear cells from chronic infiltrates gave variable staining with utr-1 antibody.

Endothelial cells and fibroblasts from various organs gave no detectable staining with either antibody (Table I).

IV. TNF-α EXPRESSION IN TISSUES

In order to obtain information on the spatial relationship of TNF-R expression and TNF production sites, TNF-α tissue expression was investigated by using mAbs. TNF-α-reactive cells were confined to the lymph follicles (Fig. 1F); within this structure the follicular dendritic cells, with their cytoplasmic projections, stained distinctly. The immune reactivity was less in the mantle zone and was almost absent in the interfollicular T cell area of the lymphoid organs. DRC staining with TNF-α was superimposable with that of htr-19 mAb. In the thymus, only a little immunoreactivity was found with TNF-α antibody, which was restricted to medullary dendritic cells. In the bone marrow, cells with monocytic morphology contained TNF-α.

To show the specificity of the immunoreactivity, incubations with TNF-α antibody were performed in the presence of excess TNF-α, which reduced the TNF-α staining. Attempts to identify cells producing lymphotoxin (TNF-β) in the tissue with two different polyclonal antibodies failed.

V. DISCUSSION

A unique distribution of the two types of TNF receptors was found in human tissues by immunohistochemistry, using two specific mAbs (8). The p55 protein, reacting with the htr-19 antibody, constituted a minor population of TNF-R, expressed in the dendritic reticulum cells of germinal centers, whereas the p75 protein recognized by the utr-1 antibody constituted the major population. These comprised interdigitating reticulum cells and activated lymphocytes in the thymic medulla and the interfollicular T cell area of lymph nodes. Based on sequential staining of serial sections and double staining, a high percentage of utr-1-positive lymphocytes and IDCs coexpress the Tac protein of the IL-2R. Tissue expression of TNF-α has been reported by McCall *et al.* (10). The TNF receptor distribution was compared with immunostaining of the same tissues, using antibody directed against TNF-α and TNF-β. The available anti-TNF-β antibodies gave no staining, but the immunoreactivity of TNF-α antibodies was strong and essentially located in the germinal center: DRCs with cell body projections into the mantle zone were stained and a few dendritic cells stained in the T cell areas. The latter results are in agreement with earlier publications (10,11).

The present data suggest that the main source of TNF-α is the macrophage-derived DRC, which also expresses the p55 TNF-R protein. In the absence of a suitable antibody, the nature of TNF-β-producing cells cannot be determined. In contrast, the p75 TNF-R sites are anatomically separated and are located mainly in the T cell areas.

Both the DRCs of germinal centers and the IDCs of the T cell areas are known to function as antigen-presenting cells and are apparently responsive to the same lymphokines. It appears that cooperation with the respective antigen-reactive lymphocytes requires a diferent receptor structure, as recognized by the utr-1 and htr-19 mAbs. The fact that activated lymphocytes coexpress receptors for IL-2 and TNF is in accordance with previous findings of p75 TNF-R expression on activated T cells (18) and supports *in vitro* observations that TNF-α plays a role in the activation of lymphocytes (12,13,22).

These results demonstrate, for the first time, a distinct distribution of the two TNF-R proteins in lymphoid tissue. In view of the differential location of cells producing and responding to this cytokine, autocrine and paracrine signaling pathways of TNF-α, which use different receptor structures, are suggested. No information is presently available as to whether the two receptor proteins also have different functions.

Investigations of pathological tissues might promote our understanding of the role of TNF-α in disease. In reactive lymph nodes, the number of p75 (utr-1)-positive cells was increased in T cell areas; epithelioid cell granulomas and giant cells in sarcoidosis expressed p75 TNF-R, suggesting a role for TNF in their formation. Experimental evidence in a parasite mouse model supports this assumption (23). Preliminary results from our laboratory revealed a high expression of p75 TNF-R on malignant lymphoma (29).

Surprisingly, the present investigation with both TNF receptor antibodies did not give any staining of endothelial cells nor of fibroblasts, smooth muscle cells, astrocytes, and oligodendrocytes, cells known to respond to TNF *in vitro* (16,17,24,27). Evidence for an important role for TNF and other cytokines in normal and pathological vascular endothelial responses and in an astonishing variety of immunopathological disease conditions (29) has been reviewed recently. The absence of immunoreactivity may be due to a low expression of receptor molecules, low sensitivity of the immunohistochemical method, or fundamental differences between cultured cells, cell lines, and the *in vitro* situation. The only TNF-R-positive cells found in nonlymphoid tissues were dendritic reticulum cells, which are located in the interstitial space of various organs, such as kidneys, lungs, and mucosae.

VI. SUMMARY

The nature and location of cells responding to tumor necrosis factor-α were investigated *in situ* by immunohistochemistry using monoclonal antibodies directed against the p75 and p55 proteins of the TNF receptor. Receptor expression was found in the thymus and secondary lymphoid tissues. In the thymus, the p75 receptor was confined to medullary lymphoblasts and dendritic cells, which costain with the Tac protein of the interleukin-2 receptor. In lymph nodes and other secondary lymphoid tissues, the p75 receptor was expressed on activated lmyphocytes and interdigitating reticulum cells of the T cell areas, whereas the p55 receptor was confined to the germinal center dendritic reticulum cells, which are the main site of TNF-α production. TNF receptor proteins were up-regulated in reactive hyperplasia together with increased TNF-α expression. Suprisingly, no TNF-R was detectable on nonlymphoid tissues. The species specificity of these TNF-antibodies was high: whereas the antibodies cross-reacted with epitopes in nonhuman primates, no immunoreactivity was detected in lower animal species, e.g., dog, rabbit, and rodents. The data presented suggest that TNF-α, which is produced by germinal center DRCs, might regulate an *in vivo* immune response through autocrine and paracrine pathways, e.g., through the p55 and p75 receptor proteins, which are expressed at different sites on the lymphoid tissue.

References

1. Old, L. J. *In* "Tumor Necrosis Factor: Structure, Mechanism of Action, Role in Disease and Therapy" (B. Bonavida and G. Granger, eds.), pp. 1–30. Karger, Basel, 1990.
2. Beutler, B., and Cerami, A. *Annu. Rev. Immunol.* **7,** 625–655 (1989).
3. Vilcek, J., and Lee, T. H. *J. Biol. Chem.* **266,** 7313–7316 (1991).
4. Pennica, D., Nedwin, G. E., Hayflick, J. S., Seeburg, P. H., Derynck, R., Palladino, M. A., Kohr, W. J., Aggarwal, B. B., and Goeddel, D. V. *Nature (London)* **312,** 724–729 (1984).
5. Old, L. J. *Science* **230,** 630–634 (1985).
6. Sung, S. J., Bjorndahl, J. M., Wong, C. Y., Kato, H. T., and Fu, S. M. *J. Exp. Med.* **167,** 937–944 (1988).
7. Amino, N., Linn, E. S., Pysher, T. J., Mier, R., Moore, G. E., and DeGroot, L. J. *J. Immunol.* **113,** 1334–1345 (1974).
8. Brockhaus, M., Schoenfeld, H. J., Schlaeger, E. J., Hunziker, W., Lesslauer, W., and Loetscher, H. *Proc. Natl. Acad. Sci. U.S.A.* **87,** 3127–3131 (1990).
9. Hohmann, H. P., Remy, R., Brockhaus, M., and van Loon, A. P. G. M. *J. Biol. Chem.* **264,** 14927–14934 (1989).

10. McCall, J. L., Kankatsu, Y., Shinsaku, F., and Parry, B. R. *Am. J. Pathol.* **135**, 421–425 (1989).

11. Ruco, L. P., Stoppacciaro, A., Donatella, P., Boraschi, D., Santoni, A., Tagliabue, A., Ucchini, S., and Baroni, C. D. *Am. J. Pathol.* **135**, 889–897 (1989).

12. Ranges, G. E., Bombara, M. P., Ramani, A. A., Rice, G. G., and Palladino, M. A. *J. Immunol.* **142**, 1203–1208 (1989).

13. Scheurich, P., Thomas, B., Ucer, U., and Pfizenmaier, K. *J. Immunol.* **138**, 1786 (1987).

14. Kehrl, J., Miller, A., and Fauci, A. *J. Exp. Med.* **166**, 786 (1987).

15. Imamura, K., Spriggs, D., and Kufe, D. *J. Immunol.* **139**, 2989–2992 (1987).

16. Lin, J. X., and Vilcek, J. *J. Biol. Chem.* **262**, 11908–11911 (1987).

17. Collins, T., Lapierre, L. A., Fiers, W., Strominger, L. J., and Pober, J. D. *Proc. Natl. Acad. Sci. U.S.A.* **83**, 446–450 (1986).

18. Dembic, Z., Loetscher, H., Gubler, U., Pan, Y. C. E., Lahm, H. W., Gentz, R., Brockhaus, M., and Lesslauer, W. *Cytokine* **2**, 231–237 (1990).

19. Loetscher, H., Pan, Y. C. E., Lahm, H. W., Gentz, R., Brockhaus, M., Tabuchi, H., and Lesslauer, W. *Cell* **61**, 351–359 (1990).

20. Schall, T. J., Lewis, M., Koller, K. J., Lee, A., Rice, G. C., Wong, G. H. E., Gatanaga, T., Granger, G. A., Lentz, R., Raab, H., Kohr, W. J., and Goeddel, D. V. *Cell* **61**, 361–370 (1990).

21. Smith, C. A., Davis, T., Anderson, D., Solam, L., Beckmann, M. P., Jerzi, R., Dower, S. K., Cosman, D., and Goodwin, R. G. *Science* **248**, 1019–1023 (1990).

22. Kuhweide, R., Van Damme, J., and Ceuppens, J. L. *Eur. J. Immunol.* **20**, 1019–1025 (1990).

23. Chensue, S. W., Otterness, I. G., Higashi, G. I., Forsch, C. S., and Kunkel, S. L. *J. Immunol.* **142**, 1281–1286 (1989).

24. Stolpen, A. H., Guinan, E. C., Fiers, W., and Pober, J. S. *Am. J. Pathol.* **123**, 16–24 (1986).

25. Warner, S. J. C., and Libby, P. *J. Immunol.* **142**, 100–109 (1989).

26. Selmaj, K. W., Farooq, M., Norton, W. T., Raine, C. S., and Brosnan, C. F. *J. Immunol.* **144**, 239 (1990).

27. Selmag, K. W., and Raine, C. S. *Ann. Neurol.* **23**, 338 (1988).

28. Pober, J. S. *Am. J. Pathol.* **133**, 426 (1988).

29. Ryffel, B., Brockhaus, M., Durrmuller, U., and Gudat, F. *Am. J. Pathol.* **139**, 7 (1991).

30. Piguet, P. F., Grau, G. E., and Vassalli, P. *Immunol. Rex.* **10**, 122, (1991).

Section III
ROLE OF CYTOKINES IN DISEASE

Tumor Necrosis Factor/ Cachectin as an Effector of T Cell- Dependent Immunopathology

Georges E. Grau, Paul-Henri Lambert, Pierre Vassalli, and Pierre-François Piguet
Department of Pathology
WHO-IRTC
University of Geneva
CH-1211 Geneva 4, Switzerland

I. INTRODUCTION

Immunopathology consists of adverse reactions generated by the immune response, classically divided into humoral and cellular (T cell-mediated)

International Review of Experimental Pathology, Volume 34B

responses. In addition, in the past few years, it has become evident that the immune system can also be expressed through the action of soluble mediators, the cytokines, which regulate the interactions not only among cells of the immune system but also between the immune system and other systems, such as components of the connective tissue (endothelial cells, fibroblasts), major metabolic pathways, or the neuroendocrine system. Cytokines have well-demonstrated roles in homeostatic mechanisms and in the defense against various infectious pathogens (1,2), but these molecules can also induce various types of lesions when produced excessively or inappropriately. One of these cytokines, tumor necrosis factor-α (TNF-α, or cachectin) appears to play a peculiar and essential role. Originally described as a factor causing hemorrhagic necrosis of tumors (3), TNF is now recognized as a cytokine with pleiotropic effects (4). This 17.5-kDa polypeptide acts as an hormone by binding to high-affinity receptors present on many or most cells of the body, leading thus to a particularly wide array of cellular responses. TNF has been involved in physiological (ontogenesis (5), thymus maturation (6,7) and physiopathological events, including several infectious, inflammatory, and immune diseases (8). The cellular sources of TNF are diverse, but the major source appears to be differentiated mononuclear phagocytes. T lymphocytes also release TNF-α and TNF-β under stimulation, and this ability might be the starting point of a number of pathologies: this is the very subject of this review. The cellular and molecular biology of TNF have been recently reviewed (9–11). The availability of recombinant material and the production of neutralizing antibodies have allowed for the appraisal of the *in vivo* relevance of TNF: Beutler, Cerami, and colleagues have demonstrated that TNF is the central endogenous mediator of the acute pathologic changes induced by bacterial lipopolysaccharides (LPS, endotoxin). Indeed, administration of recombinant TNF reproduces most of the lesions and metabolic changes observed during endotoxinemia, and LPS-induced circulatory shock and mortality are prevented by treatment with anti-TNF antibodies (12,13).

The possible implications of TNF in immunopathological reactions has been investigated only recently. It is likely that TNF is involved at several levels of the immune response. In the present review, we will concentrate first on TNF properties relevant to tissue injury, second on the role of TNF in T cell-mediated immunopathological reactions *in vivo,* and third on the possible cytokine interactions responsible for the overproduction of TNF observed in these conditions.

II. TNF PROPERTIES RELEVANT FOR IMMUNOPATHOLOGY

One of the characteristics of TNF responsible for its effects observed originally, i.e., the induction of hemorrhagic necrosis of tumors, is its numerous and potent effects on vascular endothelial cells (reviewed in refs. 14 and 15). The major effects of TNF in endotoxinemia as well as in some of the experimental models discussed below, such as cerebrovascular lesions in malaria or vascular leak in graft-versus-host disease, may indeed depend largely on the modulatory and toxic effects of TNF on endothelial cells. Another peculiar feature of TNF is its ability to induce concomitantly cellular necrosis and proliferation, which are characteristic alterations of tissue damage and remodeling observed in immunopathological reactions. *In vitro,* it has been shown that TNF, depending on the dose, can cause either proliferation (16–18) or necrosis (19–22) of various cell types. *In vivo,* administration of recombinant TNF to several species, including man, reproduces the pathological changes of gram-negative sepsis (13,23–25). A single injection of this molecule into mice induces a diffuse alveolar damage with extensive necrosis of endothelial and epithelial cells (26). In contrast, when administered in continuous subcutaneous perfusion, a broad spectrum of reactions can be reproduced, depending on the dose and duration of perfusion, ranging from proliferation of fibroblasts, deposition of collagen, and neoangiogenesis to massive tissue necrosis (27), resulting most likely from extensive endothelial cell damage. The latter type of effect is likely to involve the participation of various cell types and probably of several other cytokines.

III. POSSIBLE ROLE OF TNF IN THE IMMUNE RESPONSE

Several effects of TNF have been documented *in vitro,* such as an ability to increase T cell (28–32) and B cell (33,34) functions and a comitogenic effect in the thymocyte proliferation assay (6), and *in vivo* TNF might slightly increase the antibody response to heterologous erythrocytes. (35) Our own unpublished data, using anti-TNF antibody injections *in vivo,* do not suggest that TNF has a significant role as an immunomodulator. Injection of anti-TNF antibody in mice did not affect an *in vivo* mixed leukocyte reaction (MLR) (36), whereas it suppressed a MLR *in vitro* (37). In addition, this antibody had no effect *in vivo* on IgM or IgG antibody responses to heterologous erythrocytes, neither in primary nor in secondary responses, and in mice undergoing collagen arthritis did not affect the humoral response to bovine type II collagen (38). However, more recently, it has been established that repeated injections of TNF into normal mice leads to a progressive diminution of cell-mediated immune responses *in vivo,* the humoral responses remaining unchanged (39). Therefore, the precise role of TNF in the immune response may rest on a delicate balance that is poorly understood, but possibly affecting cellular rather than humoral responses.

IV. IMMUNOPATHOLOGICAL REACTIONS INVOLVING T LYMPHOCYTES AND TNF

Table I summarizes the findings observed in models of immunopathological reactions. Besides shock induced by endotoxin, which is unrelated to T cells, these comprise infectious diseases (malaria and *Mycobacterium bovis* infection), immune-mediated pathological reactions such as graft-versus-host-disease (GVHD), and a drug-induced immunopathological reaction, the alveolar damage and fibrosis elicited by bleomycin. Although they may appear to be completely unrelated in their course and histopathological appearance, the epression of these diseases requires both T lymphocytes and TNF.

Experimental cerebral malaria triggered by *Plasmodium berghei* Anka infection is characterized by a neurological syndrome associated with circulatory shock and death occurring in about 85% of the mice, irrespective of their level of parasitemia. The main lesion is a sequestration of leukocytes in the brain venulae, leading to a hemorrhagic necrosis (40). Graft-versus-host-disease is produced by the transfer of foreign T lymphocytes into an immunocompromised host, which leads to cachexia and death over the following weeks. The main lesions in the acute phase of GVHD are isolated focal epithelial cell necrosis in the epidermis, the gut mucosa (36), and the alveolar epithelium (42), accompanied by vascular leak (41), and dyshemopoiesis. These lesions resemble those observed during some immune or

Table I. Evidence for a Role for TNF in Various Immunopathological Reactions

Model	T lymphocyte dependency	TNF production		Events prevented by anti-TNF antibody
		Serum	Organs	
Endotoxin shock	−	+	+	Tissue lesions, mortality [13,23]
Cerebral malaria	+	+	+	Mortality, cerebrovascular damage, macrophage accumulation [40]
GVHD	+	−	+	Mortality, cachexia epithelial and intestinal damage, dysmyelopoiesis [36,42]
BCG infection	+	−	+	Macrophage accumulation, formation of bactericidal granulomas [43]
Pulmonary fibrosis (bleomycin)	+	−	+	Collagen deposition, alveolar damage [44]

autoimmune diseases. Inoculation of *M. bovis* (bacillus Calmette and Guérin, or BCG) into susceptible mice leads to a dissemination of the mycobacteria associated with the accumulation, growth, and differentiation of macrophages organized in disseminated granulomas (43), in the macrophages of which the mycobacteria are progressively eliminated. Bleomycin pneumopathy is induced by the intratracheal instillation of 0.1 U of bleomycin into susceptible mice. The main lesions observed after 7 days are necrosis of alveolar endothelial and epithelial cells, growth of fibroblasts, and collagen deposition (44). It is considered as a model for human idiopathic pulmonary fibrosis.

A. Diseases Associated with TNF Overproduction

An increase of TNF production can be demonstrated by an increased serum TNF level, as observed during endotoxinemia (12). In malaria-infected mice, serum TNF concentrations appear and acutely rise at the time of the neurological syndrome. Interestingly, this association has also been found in humans: high plasma TNF levels correlate with disease severity in children with severe *Plasmodium falciparum* malaria, and particularly with cerebral malaria (45,46). The relationship between experimental and human cerebral malaria has been recently reviewed (47). In our other experimental models, however, an elevation of serum TNF level is not detectable, but local TNF overproduction is evidenced by an increased TNF mRNA accumulation in the RNA extracted from affected organs, or at the site of lesions, as observed, for instance, during GVHD (36), bleomycin pneumopathy (44), or BCG infection (wherein the diffuse presence of TNF within epithelioid cells of the granulomas is detectable by immunofluorescence) (43).

B. Pathological Manifestations Abrogated by Anti-TNF Antibody

The injection of 1–2 mg/week of a rabbit antimurine TNF-α IgG preparation prevents mortality as well as most of the pathological manifestations of these diseases (Table I), with the exception of BCG granulomas. In this condition, the lack of well-differentiated granulomas resulting from anti-TNF antibody injections leads to progressive growth of BCG, which eventually kills the animals. In malaria, it should be noted that rabbit anti-TNF antibody treatment does not interfere with the course of infection with malaria parasites (40) and does not inhibit T lymphocyte activation and proliferation *in vivo* (36), thus indicating that TNF is not involved during the sensitization phase, but rather during the effector phase of the immune response. This appears to be true in BCG infection, when anti-TNF antibody injections are started after granuloma appearance (43). A membrane form of TNF on some lymphocytes (48) has been recently described, but for the reasons just mentioned it does not appear that the effect of anti-TNF antibody injection results simply from the elimination of TNF-bearing T lymphocytes.

C. Requirement of T Lymphocytes for Lesions and TNF Overproduction

Treatment of malaria-infected mice with anti-CD4 monoclonal antibody depletes these mice in the $CD4^+$ T lymphocyte subset and prevents elevation of the serum TNF level and the associated lethal neurovascular lesions (40,49). Conversely, thymectomized mice are resistant to the development of cerebral malaria but are rendered susceptible to this lethal complication when selectively reconstituted with $CD4^+$ T cells (49). The development of GVHD requires T lymphocytes for both the expression of the disease (50) and the overproduction of TNF (36,42). Indeed, the transfer into irradiated semiallogeneic recipient mice of parental T lymphocytes and bone marrow cells, but not of T-depleted bone marrow cells alone, leads to morbidity associated with an elevation of the TNF mRNA level (36,42). During infection with *M. bovis,* the macrophage accumulation and differentiation resulting in granuloma formation can be abrogated by depletion of T lymphocytes (51). Also, BCG infection in athymic nude mice cannot give rise to well-formed, protective granulomas. The pulmonary fibrosis of bleomycin-induced pneumopathy cannot be elicited in nude mice (52) or in mice depleted *in vivo* of $CD4^+$ T lymphocytes, which show no elevation of lung TNF mRNA levels (44).

V. INDUCTION AND CELLULAR ORIGIN OF TNF

T lymphocytes are capable of producing both TNF-α (or cachectin) and TNF-β (or lymphotoxin) *in vitro* (53). It is, however, uncertain whether their contribution is quantitatively important because, in the models listed in Table I, T lymphocytes are much less abundant in the lesions than are macrophages. Particularly, the role of lymphotoxin in lesions remains to be investigated because it is not produced by macrophages. TNF-β mRNA is not detectable at a level comparable to that of TNF-α in the affected tissues (unpublished observations). Because macrophages can produce much larger quantities of TNF than can T lymphocytes (10), it is therefore more likely that the main effect of T lymphocytes is to increase TNF-α production in macrophages and other leukocytes by the secretion of cytokines. Several T lymphocyte-derived cytokines are capable of either increasing the number of TNF-producing macrophages, or their activation for TNF secretion. In order to determine the respective role of the T cell-derived cytokines, we have attempted to block selectively their activity *in vivo* by injecting neutralizing monospecific antibodies.

A. Granulocyte–Macrophage Colony-Stimulating Factor and Interleukin-3

We have observed that injection or perfusion of recombinant granulocyte–macrophage colony-stimulating factor (GM-CSF) and IL-3 into mice are capable of increasing TNF mRNA levels in various organs, including lung and liver (P. F. Piguet *et al.,* unpublished observations). Involvement of these cytokines can be demonstrated directly in the cerebral malaria model: a combined treatment with antibodies against GM-CSF and IL-3 prevents the accumulation of macrophages in large numbers, as well as the elevation of serum TNF levels and mortality due to the cerebral syndrome (54). In the GVHD model, these antibodies decrease mortality and prevent epithelial damage (P. F. Piguet, unpublished observations). In contrast, we have never been able to significantly alter BCG granuloma formation by injection of antibodies to IL-3 and GM-CSF, perhaps because it is the increase in TNF that, by mechanisms of autoamplification, is essential to the development of the granuloma (43) (see below).

B. Interferon-γ

In vitro, IFN-γ can increase TNF transcription by macrophages (55), but whether this also requires trace amounts of LPS is not clear. *In vivo,* IFN-γ seems to either enhance or inhibit immunopathological reactions such as adjuvant arthritis (56) or allergic encephalomyelitis (57). In the cerebral malaria model, antimurine IFN-γ monoclonal antibody treatment prevents mortality and elevation of the serum TNF level (58), but does so, as opposed to anti-IL-3 and anti-GM-CSF antibodies, without decreasing macrophage infiltration into lymphoid tissues. This is compatible with a role of IFN-γ in macrophage activation rather than in their accumulation. In GVHD, however, we found that *in vivo* administration of these antibodies acceler-ates the disease (P. F. Piguet *et al.,* unpublished observations). This might be related to the general effect of IFN-γ on cell proliferation, which can de-crease the expansion of donor T cells. We found that bleomycin-induced fibrosis can be attenuated by IFN-γ or aggravated by anti-IFN-γ antibodies (P. F. Piguet *et al.,* unpublished observations). IFN-γ has been reported to decrease collagen synthesis by fibroblasts. There is little doubt that, in addition to its stimulation of TNF secretion, IFN-γ has several other activities: its global effect *in vivo* is therefore difficult to predict.

C. Interleukin-2

When infused into mice, this cytokine markedly increases the number of large granular leukocytes (LGLs) as well as the TNF mRNA levels in various organs (ref. 59 and unpublished observations). In contrast to *in vitro* conditions, IL-2 infusion does not increase the number of T lymphocytes *in vivo* (59). Because IL-2 increases TNF production in both LGLs and macrophages *in vitro,* it is therefore likely that LGLs too may be involved *in vivo* in TNF release in some conditions. Consistent with this view is our observation that cells with features of LGLs are sequestered in brain capillaries and venules during experimental cerebral malaria (G. E. Grau *et al.,* unpublished observations). GVHD as well as bleomycin pneumopathy can be abrogated by anti-IL-2 antibodies (ref. 60 and unpublished observations); this effect might be due in part to prevention of the IL-2-induced enhancement of TNF secretion, and to expansion of the T cells. The possible pathways leading to an inappropriately high TNF production *in vivo* are represented schematically in Fig. 1.

D. TNF

TNF in some circumstances strongly promotes the accumulation and differentiation of macrophages, which are then induced to produce more TNF. *In vitro,* incubation of macrophages with TNF increases TNF mRNA levels (43,61). *In vivo,* as a result of anti-TNF antibody treatment, the infiltration of lymphoid tissues by macrophages during cerebral malaria is markedly reduced (40), and the level of TNF mRNA is strikingly diminished in BCG granulomas (43). Because TNF is a strong inducer of GM-CSF release by endothelial cells and fibroblasts, it may also act *in vivo* through a variety of indirect mechanisms. It is important to point out that TNF released by stimulated T lymphocytes up-regulates the expression of cell adhesion molecules on endothelial cells of some venules. This promotes the venular adhesion of leukocytes through their corresponding ligands (e.g., LFA-1, Mac-1) and thus will favor the progressive development of local tissue inflammatory

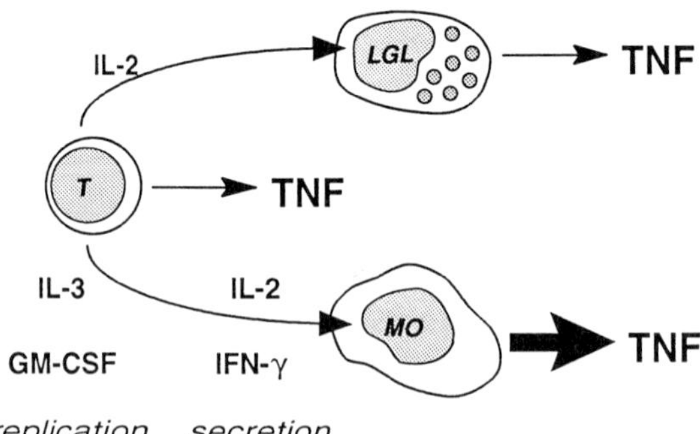

Fig. 1. Schematic representation of the possible pathways possibly involved in inappropriately high TNF production *in vivo*. LGL, Large granular lymphocyte; MO, mononuclear phagocyte.

cell infiltration, including cells producing more TNF. This may explain why anti-TNF antibody treatment prevents the focal arrest of leukocytes in brain and lung vessels during cerebral malaria. Interestingly, we have recently shown that anti-LFA-1 monoclonal antibody treatment prevents cerebral malaria (62).

VI. CONCLUSIONS

A. TNF Is an Effector of Tissue Damage

We have reviewed various types of pathological alterations that (1) are associated with an increased TNF production, (2) are abrogated by *in vivo* administration of anti-TNF antibody, and (3) resemble in some cases lesions induced by TNF perfusion. It is therefore likely that TNF is an effector of these tissue reactions or damage. It should be stressed that it is only when the production of TNF becomes inappropriate that this cytokine is able to cause tissue injury. One of the mechanisms that can account for TNF overproduction is the triggering of a cascade of T cell-derived cytokines, as demonstrated in experimental cerebral malaria: on the one hand, IL-3 and GM-CSF act by enlarging the macrophage pool in lymphoid organs, and on the other hand, IFN-γ activates these macrophages to release excess amounts of TNF (47). In contrast, when its production remains well tuned, TNF plays a major role in the defense against infections, including malaria. In BCG infection, the high levels of TNF produced remain localized within each granuloma and enter the blood only if the animals are exposed to LPS (3,43). Along this line, the implication of TNF in the BCG granuloma model illustrates particularly well its duality: TNF is a crucial element in the limitation of *M. bovis* expansion, but is also the cytokine through which tissue lesions occur (granulomas and associated liver damage). This is a typical example of immunopathology. In this case, pathology can be seen as the price to pay for the beneficial effects of TNF.

B. Activation of T Lymphocytes Is Likely to Raise TNF Levels

In four different immunopathological reactions elicited by T lymphocytes, these cells are required for TNF overproduction, it is likely that in a wide variety of conditions resulting in an activation of the T lymphocytes, such as infectious or autoimmune diseases, the activation of the immune system will also lead to an increase in TNF production. Numerous recent reports have indeed documented the association between autoimmune diseases and TNF overproduction. High brain TNF mRNA levels have been described in multiple sclerosis (63). In MRL-*lpr/lpr* mice, a striking constitutive high level of

TNF mRNA expression has been found in the abnormal subpopulation of CD4$^-$ CD8$^-$ lymphocytes that accumulate in lymphoid organs (64). Also, freshly isolated and unstimulated renal glomeruli of these mice spontaneously release TNF (and IL-1 β) *in vitro* when signs of lupus nephritis become evident (65). Glomerular macrophages and mesangial cells, which are prominent in mouse autoimmune nephritis, represent the local source of the released TNF (65). Kupffer cells isolated from the liver of these mice also spontaneously release TNF *in vitro* (66). Comparable results of detectable TNF mRNA in renal cortex, increasing with age and when signs of glomerular disease become conspicuous, have been obtained in (NZB $\times$ NZW)F$_1$ hybrid mice (67). It must be stressed, however, that autoimmune-prone mice produce the lowest TNF levels (in response to various stimuli) known so far (68). Thus, the balance between local TNF production and constitutive capacity to release this cytokine appears critical in autoimmunity. In an *in vivo* model of direct T cell activation induced by antimurine CD3 mAb, it has been shown that most of the pathological changes observed are attributable to TNF (69). Likewise, serum concentrations of TNF and other cytokines are elevated in patients receiving OKT3 mAb (70,71).

C. TNF Has a Central Role in T Lymphocyte-Induced Immunopathological Reactions

The observations discussed here widen the scope of T cell-mediated reactions, because, in addition to the classical reactions of cell-mediated lympholysis (CML) or delayed-type hypersensitivity (DTH), TNF released by activated T cells might also be involved in these reactions in an autocrine or paracrine manner, or even have far-reaching (i.e., hormonelike) influences on nonimmunocompetent cells. These notions may thus improve the understanding of lesions observed during immunopathological reactions, which were underestimated in the classical studies. One example is cachexia (i.e., the acute loss of hypodermic fat) observed during chronic infectious diseases or GVHD, which appears to be T cell dependent. Other examples are necrosis of various cell types, which is observed within epithelia during GVHD, or in the brain vessel walls during cerebral malaria, and the fibrosis observed in T cell-dependent bleomycin pneumopathy. Finally, one of the potentially essential mechanisms of action of TNF released by T lymphocytes is the up-regulation of cell adhesion molecules, or "addressins," on venular endothelial cells (72). This favors the tissue migration of various types of leukocytes, which participate in, and possibly amplify, the inflammatory infiltrate. All these very diverse pathological changes are best understood if related to the diffusion of a mediator with multiple properties.

Acknowledgments

This work was supported by grants from the World Bank/United Nations Development Program/World Health Organization, Special Programme for Training and Research in Tropical Diseases (No. 870107 to G. E. G.), Swiss National Science Foundation (No. 32-28822-90 to G. E. G. and 3.650.0.87 to P. V.), and by the Sandoz Research Foundation. G. E. G. is supported by the Cloëtta Foundation, Zürich, Switzerland. The expert technical assistance of D. Gretener, C. Gysler, and C. Vesin is gratefully acknowledged.

References

1. Blanchard, D. K., Djeu, J. Y., Klein, T. W., Friedman, H., and Stewart, W. E. *J. Leukocyte Biol.* **43**, 429–435 (1988).
2. Clark, I. A., Hunt, N. H., Butcher, G. A., and Cowden, W. B. *J. Immunol.* **139**, 3493–3496 (1987).
3. Carswell, E. A., Old, L. J., Kassel, R. L., Green, S., Fiore, N., and Williamson, B. *Proc. Natl. Acad. Sci. U.S.A.* **72**, 3666–3670 (1975).
4. Beutler, B., and Cerami, A. *N. Engl. J. Med.* **316**, 379–385 (1987).
5. Yamasu, K., Onoe, H., Soma, G., Oshima, H., and Mizuno, D. *J. Biol. Response Modif.* **8**, 644–655 (1989).
6. Ranges, G. E., Zlotnik, A., Espevik, T., Dinarello, C. A., Cerami, A., and Palladino, M. A., Jr. *J. Exp. Med.* **167**, 1472–1478 (1988).
7. Suda, T., Murray, R., Fischer, M., Yokota, T., and Zlotnik, A. *J. Immunol.* **144**, 1783–1787 (1990).
8. Tracey, K. J., Vlassara, H., and Cerami, A. *Lancet* **1**, 1122–1126 (1989).
9. Le, J., and Vilcek, J. *Lab. Invest.* **561**, 234–238 (1987).
10. Beutler, B., and Cerami, A. *Annu. Rev. Biochem.* **57**, 505–518 (1988).
11. Raine, C. S., and Cross, A. H. *Lab. Invest.* **62**, 133–134 (1990).
12. Beutler, B., Milsark, I. W., and Cerami, A. C. *Science* **229**, 869–871 (1985).
13. Tracey, K. J., Beutler, B., Lowry, S. F., *et al. Science* **234**, 470–474 (1986).
15. Cotran, R. S., and Pober, J. S. *Kidney Int.* **35**, 969–975 (1989).
16. Suzuki, K., Hara, M., Kitani, A., *et al. Biochim. Biophys. Acta* **1042**, 352–358 (1990).
17. Selmaj, K. W., Farooq, M., Norton, W. T., Raine, C. S., and Brosnan, C. F. *J. Immunol.* **144**, 129–135 (1990).
18. Branch, D. R., Turner, A. R., and Larry, L. J. *Blood* **73**, 307–311 (1989).
19. Ruff, M. R., and Gifford, G. E. *J. Immunol.* **125**, 1671–1677 (1980).
20. Peck, R., Brockhaus, M., and Frey, J. R. *Cell. Immunol.* **122**, 1–10 (1989).
21. Selmaj, K. W., and Raine, C. S. *Ann. Neurol.* **23**, 338–346 (1988).
22. Taverne, J., Rayner, D. C., van der Meide, P. H., Lydyard, P. M., Bidey, S. P., and Cooke, A. *Eur. J. Immunol.* **17**, 1855–1858 (1987).
23. Tracey, K. J., Fong, Y., Hesse, D. G., *et al. Nature (London)* **330**, 662–664 (1987).
24. Johnson, J., Meyrick, B., Jesmok, G., and Brigham, K. L. *J. Appl. Physiol.* **66**, 1448–1454 (1989).
25. Michie, H. R., Spriggs, D. R., Manogue, K. R., *et al. Surgery* **104**, 280–286 (1988).
26. Talmadge, J. E., Bowersox, O., Tribble, H., Lee, S. H., Shepard, H. M., and Liggit, D. *Am. J. Pathol.* **128**, 410–424 (1987).
27. Piguet, P. F., Grau, G. E., and Vassalli, P. *Am. J. Pathol.* **136**, 103–110 (1990).
28. Plaetinck, G., Declercq, W., Tavernier, J., Nabholz, M., and Fiers, W. *Eur. J. Immunol.* **17**, 1835–1838 (1987).

29. Nakano, K., Okugawa, K., Furuichi, H., Matsui, Y., and Sohmura, Y. *Cell. Immunol.* **120,** 154–164 (1989).

30. Shimamoto, Y., Pichyangkul, S., and Khan, A. *Proc. Soc. Exp. Biol. Med.* **189,** 310–316 (1988).

31. Talmadge, J. E., Phillips, H., Schneider, M., *et al. Cancer Res.* **48,** 544–550 (1988).

32. Lin, H. Y., Davis, P. J., Davis, F. B., Chadha, K. C., and Thacore, H. R. *J. Interferon Res.* **10,** 39–46 (1990).

33. Jelinek, D. F., and Lipsky, P. E. *J. Immunol.* **139,** 2970–2976 (1987).

34. Kehrl, J. H., Miller, A., and Fauci, A. S. *J. Exp. Med.* **166,** 786–791 (1987).

35. Ghiara, P., Boraschi, D., Nencioni, L., Ghezzi, P., and Tagliabue, A. *J. Immunol.* **139,** 3676–3679 (1987).

36. Piguet, P. F., Grau, G. E., Allet, B., and Vassalli, P. *J. Exp. Med.* **166,** 1280–1289 (1987).

37. Shalaby, M. R., Espevik, T., Rice, G. C., *et al. J. Immunol.* **141,** 499–503 (1988).

38. Piguet, P. F., *et al.* Submitted (1990).

39. Gordon, C., and Wofsy, D. *J. Immunol.* **144,** 1753–1758 (1990).

40. Grau, G. E., Fajardo, L. F., Piguet, P. F., Allet, B., Lambert, P. H., and Vassalli, P. *Science* **237,** 1210–1212 (1987).

41. Dumler, J. S., Beschorner, W. E., Farmer, E. R., Di Gennaro, K. A., Saral, R., and Santos, G. W. *Am. J. Pathol.* **135,** 1097–1103 (1989).

42. Piguet, P. F., Grau, G. E., Collart, M. A., Vassalli, P., and Kapanci, Y. *Lab. Invest.* **61,** 37–45 (1989).

43. Kindler, V., Sappino, A. P., Grau, G. E., Piguet, P. F., and Vassalli, P. *Cell* **56,** 731–740 (1989).

44. Piguet, P. F., Collart, M. A., Grau, G. E., Kapanci, Y., and Vassalli, P. *J. Exp. Med.* **170,** 655–663 (1989).

45. Grau, G. E., Taylor, T. E., Molyneux, M. E., *et al. N. Engl. J. Med.* **320,** 1586–1591 (1989).

46. Kern, P., Hemmer, C. J., Vandamme, J., Gruss, H. J., and Dietrich, M. *Am. J. Med.* **87,** 139–143 (1989).

47. Grau, G. E., Piguet, P. F., Vassalli, P., and Lambert, P. H. *Immunol. Rev.* **112,** 49–70 (1989).

48. Kinkhabwala, M., Sehajpal, P., Sklonik, E., *et al. J. Exp. Med.* **171,** 941–946 (1990).

49. Grau, G. E., Piguet, P. F., Engers, H. D., Louis, J. A., Vassalli, P., and Lambert, P. H. *J. Immunol.* **137,** 2348–2354 (1986).

50. Korngold, R., and Sprent, J. *J. Exp. Med.* **148,** 1687–1698 (1978).

51. Ando, M., Dannenberg, A. M., and Shima, K. *J. Immunol.* **109,** 8–19 (1972).

52. Schrier, D. J., Phan, S. H., and McGarry, B. M. *Am. Rev. Respir. Dis.* **127,** 614–617 (1983).

53. Cuturi, M. C., Murphy, M., Costa-Giomi, M. P., Weinmann, R., Perussia, B., and Trinchieri, G. *J. Exp. Med.* **165,** 1581–1594 (1987).

54. Grau, G. E., Kindler, V., Piguet, P. F., Lambert, P. H., and Vassalli, P. *J. Exp. Med.* **168,** 1499–1504 (1988).

55. Collart, M. A., Belin, D., Vassalli, J. D., Dekossodo, S., and Vassalli, P. *J. Exp. Med.* **163,** 2113–2118 (1986).

56. Jacob, C. J., Holoshitz, J., Van der Meide, P., Strober, S., and McDevitt, H. O. *J. Immunol.* **142,** 1500–1505 (1989).

57. Billiau, A., Heremans, H., Vandekerckhove, F., *et al. J. Immunol.* **140,** 1506–1510 (1988).

58. Grau, G. E., Heremans, H., Piguet, P. F., *et al. Proc. Natl. Acad. Sci. U.S.A.* **86,** 5572–5574 (1989).

59. Piguet, P. F., Grau, G. E., Irle, C., and Vassalli, P. *Eur. J. Immunol.* **16,** 1257–1261 (1986).

60. Ferrara, J. L., Marion, A., McIntyre, J. F., Murphy, G. F., and Burakoff, S. J. *J. Immunol.* **137,** 1874–1877 (1986).

61. Philip, R., and Epstein, L. B. *Nature (London)* **323,** 86–89 (1986).

62. Grau, G. E., Pointaire, P., Piguet, P. F., *et al. Eur. J. Immunol.* **21,** 2265–2267 (1991).

63. Hofman, F. M., Hinton, D. R., Johnson, K., and Merrill, J. E. *J. Exp. Med.* **170,** 607–612 (1989).

64. Murray, L., and Martens, C. *Eur. J. Immunol.* **19,** 563–565 (1989).

65. Boswell, J. M., Yui, M. A., Burt, D. W., and Kelley, V. E. *J. Immunol.* **141,** 3850–3857 (1988).

66. Magilavy, D. B., and Rothstein, J. L. *J. Exp. Med.* **168,** 789–794 (1988).

67. Brennan, D. C., Yui, M. A., Wuthrich, R. P., and Kelley, V. E. *J. Immunol.* **143,** 3470–3475 (1989).

68. Jacob, C. O., and McDevitt, H. O. *Nature (London)* **331,** 356–358 (1988).

69. Ferran, C., Sheehan, K. C., Dy, M., *et al. Eur. J. Immunol.* **20,** 509–515 (1990).

70. Chatenoud, L., Ferran, C., Reuter, A., *et al. N. Engl. J. Med.* **320,** 1420–1421 (1989).

71. Abramowicz, D., Schandene, L., Goldman, M., *et al. Transplantation* **47,** 606–608 (1989).

72. Berg, E. L., Goldstein, L. A., Jutila, M. A., *et al. Immunol. Rev.* **108,** 5–18 (1989).

Cytokines Involved in Pulmonary Fibrosis

Pierre-François Piguet
Département de Pathologie
Université de Genève
CH-1211 Genève 4, Switzerland

I. INTRODUCTION

Numerous pulmonary diseases cause pulmonary fibrosis, leading eventually
to respiratory insufficiency. As a group, pulmonary diseases are responsible
for about 4% of human deaths (Bitterman and Henke, 1991). Among the
etiologies are drugs, pulmonary hypertension, autoimmune diseases and
inhalation of nondegradable particles (Colby and Churg, 1986). Pulmonary
fibrosis is characterized by an alteration of the alveolar septa associated with
growth of interstitial cells and accumulation of various proteins of the
extracellular matrix (Bowden, 1987). Such tissue remodeling implies complex interactions between cells of the alveolar septa (i.e., endothelial, epithelial, and interstitial cells) and leukocytes, which are mediated by cytokines
and other mediators. In this review the focus will be on the role of cytokines
in experimental pulmonary fibrosis induced in mice by bleomycin or dust
particles, and various other types of pulmonary fibrosis, such as idiopathic
pulmonary fibrosis and sarcoidosis.

International Review of Experimental Pathology, Volume 34B

II. FIBROGENIC CYTOKINES PRODUCED DURING PULMONARY FIBROSIS

A. Fibrogenic Cytokines

Fibrogenesis can result from an increase in the growth of fibroblasts, an increase in the rate of collagen synthesis, or a decrease in the rate of collagen degradation. Cytokines that are known to modulate these responses *in vitro* or *in vivo* are listed in Table I.

In vitro fibroblast studies are complicated by the heterogeneity of fibroblast cell lines, which may exhibit opposite types of responsiveness. These variable responses possibly correspond to different fibroblast subpopulations existing *in vivo*, which have been reported to differ in their expression of different surface proteins (Phipps *et al.*, 1990), α-actin content (Sappino *et al.*, 1990), and responses to growth factors (Goldring *et al.*, 1990). Thus, interstitial cells that accumulate during bleomycin- or silica-induced fibrosis differ in their content of α-actin, with bleomycin inducing α-actin-positive cells (Mitchell *et al.*, 1989) and silicosis inducing α-actin-negative cells (P. F. Piguet, unpublished observations). In addition, opposing conclusions might emerge from the exploration of cytokines *in vitro* or *in vivo*; e.g., tumor necrosis factor (TNF) is commonly considered to be antifibrogenic because it increases the collagenolytic activity of cell lines (Dayer *et al.*, 1985), but following infusion into mice, TNF is strongly fibrogenic, increasing both the growth of fibroblasts and collagen deposition, either locally or within the lung (Piguet *et al.*, 1990a,b).

Several cytokines are known or suspected to be fibrogenic. Interleukin-1 (IL-1) is a highly pleiotropic cytokine that exists in two forms, IL-1-α and IL-1-β; both forms are around 17 kDa (reviewed in Dinarello, 1989). IL-1 is mitogenic for some fibroblast lines (Schmidt *et al.*, 1982; Thornton *et al.*, 1990) and can, depending on the cell line, either increase the synthesis or the degradation of collagen (Matsushima *et al.*, 1985; Postlethwaite *et al.*, 1983).

Table I. Cytokines that Influence Growth of Fibroblasts and Collagen Secretion

Cytokine	Fibroblast proliferation	Collagen secretion	Fibrogenesis *in vivo*
IL-1	+/−	+/−	
TNF-α	+/−	+/−	+
TGF-β	+/−	+	+
FGF	+		+
PDGF	+	+	+
IFN-γ	−	−	−

Tumor necrosis factor is a pleiotropic cytokine, initially isolated on the basis of its capacity to induce tumor necrosis (Beutler and Cerami, 1988). It exists in two forms, TNF-α and TNF-β, both having molecular masses around 17 kDa. TNF has a wide range of biological activities, including fibrogenic activity; *in vitro,* it enhances the proliferation of some fibroblast lines but inhibits others (Sugarman *et al.,* 1985) and it inhibits collagen secretion (Dayer *et al.,* 1985). *In vivo,* it is strongly fibrogenic (Piguet *et al.,* 1990a,b).

Transforming growth factor-β (TGF-β) corresponds to a family of disulfide-linked homodimers (Wahl *et al.,* 1989). It is produced by many cell types and may be involved in various biological processes, notably development, wound healing, and immune response. It may enhance the proliferation of some fibroblast lines *in vitro* but inhibits others (Thornton *et al.,* 1990); it increases their rate of collagen secretion (Roberts *et al.,* 1986) and is fibrogenic *in vivo* (Roberts and Sporn, 1989; Roberts *et al.,* 1986; Sprugel *et al.,* 1987).

Platelet-derived growth factor (PDGF) was initially isolated from platelets but is now known to be produced by various cells (Ross *et al.,* 1986). It exists in several forms and is made of homo- and heterodimers of about 30 kDa. It has been reported to enhance the replication of fibroblasts and the rate of collagen secretion and to be fibrogenic *in vivo* (Thornton *et al.,* 1990). Its production has been reported in association with idiopathic pulmonary fibrosis (Antoniades *et al.,* 1990).

Fibroblast growth factors (FGFs) comprise a family of peptides with a potent fibrogenic activity *in vitro* and *in vivo* (Sprugel *et al.,* 1987) but whose biological role is poorly understood (reviewed in Rifkin and Moscatelli, 1989; Klagsbrun and Edelman, 1989). They are present in a wide variety of cell types but it is not established whether their synthesis and secretion are regulated and/or if they are released only by damaged cells (D'Amore, 1990).

The data in Table I are certainly not complete and there are other cytokines that are fibrogenic *in vivo,* perhaps as a result of the activation of other factors, notably IL-2 and GM-CSF.

Interferon-γ is known to inhibit collagen secretion and the growth of various cells (including fibroblasts) (Rosenbloom *et al.,* 1984). It is an antifibrogenic agent that has been used successfully *in vivo* (Hyde *et al.,* 1988).

B. Methodological Considerations for Evaluation of Cytokine Production

An increase in cytokine production during fibrotic reactions suggests involvement of cytokines in disease processes. This can be explored using different methods: (1) Tissue extraction is obviously the most direct approach and has been performed successfully for TGF-β during bleomycin-induced pulmonary fibrosis (Khalil *et al.,* 1989). (2) RNA extraction and evaluation of the mRNA content by Northern blotting have been performed for several cytokines, including IL-1, TNF, TGF, and PDGF; the main limitation of these processes results from the possibility that differences in the mRNA levels will not necessarily correlate with differences in the amounts of proteins produced, because of posttranscriptional regulation of protein production. (3) Another approach is isolation and exploration of cellular components; alveolar leukocytes and macrophages, freshly prepared or after culture, have been extensively explored in the context of pulmonary fibrosis, an approach that is based on the assumption that these cells are representative, quantitatively or qualitatively, of cytokine production within the lung. However, the epithelium or the interstice might be an important source of some of the fibrogenic cytokines, such as PDGF and TGF-β. Furthermore, cytokines such as TNF, delivered to the alveolar space, do not appear to affect the interstice (Fuchs *et al.,* 1990).

C. Pulmonary Fibrosis and Fibrogenic Cytokine Production

Correlations or the absence of correlations between cytokine production and pulmonary fibrosis are summarized on Table II. In our studies, based on the evaluation of the mRNA levels of various cytokines, the best correlations are observed with TNF-α, whose mRNA shows a 10- to 80-fold long-lasting increase in correlation with either bleomycin or silica-induced fibrosis (Piguet *et al.,* 1989, 1990a). The mRNA of other fibrogenic cytokines shows only a transient and moderate (two- to threefold) change during these reactions.

D. Effects of Cytokines and Anticytokine Agents

Correlations do not establish a causal relationship between cytokine overproduction and fibrogenic reaction. More direct information can be obtained with the use of inhibitors. Anticytokine antibodies have been used with success in various conditions (Piguet *et al.,* 1991a), but more recently, inhibitors made with the extracellular portion of the receptor or with receptor antagonists have been explored (Fanslow *et al.,* 1990; Lesslauer *et al.,* 1991). Table III summarizes studies performed *in vivo* using cytokine or anticytokine agents. It is evident that this type of evaluation is incomplete at this time, as potent inhibitors are not available for all potentially fibrogenic cytokines.

Table II. Correlation between Pulmonary Fibrosis and Cytokine Overproduction

Model	Cytokine	Method[a]	Correlation[b]	Ref.
Experimental bleomycin	TGF-β	TE	+	Khalil *et al.* (1989)
	TGF-β	RNA	+	Piguet *et al.* (1989)
	PDGF	RNA	+	Piguet (1992)
	IL-1	RNA	−	Piguet *et al.* (1989)
		AM	+	Suwabe *et al.* (1988)
	TNF	RNA	+	Piguet *et al.* (1989)
Experimental silicosis	TGF-β	RNA	−	Piguet *et al.* (1990a)
	PDGF	RNA	−	Piguet (1992)
	IL-1	RNA	−	Piguet *et al.* (1990a)
	TNF	RNA	+	Piguet *et al.* (1989)
		AM	+	Bissonnette *et al.* (1989)
Experimental asbestosis	PDGF	AM	+	Bauman *et al.* (1987)
	IL-1	AM	+	Lemaire (1991)
	TNF-α	AM	+	Bissonnette *et al.* (1989)
Pneumoconiosis	TNF-α	AM	+	Lassalle *et al.* (1990)
	IL-1	AM	+	Lassalle *et al.* (1990)
Idiopathic pulmonary fibrosis	IL-1	AM	−	Rochemonteix-Galve *et al.* (1990)
	TNF	AM	−	Rochemonteix-Galve *et al.* (1990)
	PDGF	RNA	+	Antoniades *et al.* (1990)
Sarcoidosis	IL-1	AM	−	Rochemonteix-Galve *et al.* (1990)
	TNF	AM	−	Rochemonteix-Galve *et al.* (1990)
	IL-1	AM	+	Hunninghake (1984)
	TNF	AM	+	Spatafora *et al.* (1989)

[a] TE, Evaluation of the cytokine by tissue extraction; AM, studies of the alveolar macrophages *ex vivo* or after culture; RNA, evaluation of the mRNA in the RNA extracted from whole lung.

[b] A + indicates a positive correlation; −, negative or absence of a correlation between disease and cytokine production.

Table III. Modulation of Experimental Pulmonary Fibrosis by Cytokines or Anticytokines

Cytokine or antagonist[a]	Model	Effect	Ref.
TNF	Bleomycin	Aggravation	Piguet *et al.* (1991a)
TNF	Silicosis	Aggravation	Piguet *et al.* (1990)
TNF antagonist	Bleomycin	Protection	Piguet *et al.* (1989)
TNF antagonist	Silicosis	Protection	Piguet *et al.* (1990)
IFN-γ	Bleomycin	Protection	Hyde *et al.* (1988)
IFN-γ antagonist	Bleomycin	Aggravation	P. F. Piguet (unpublished observations)
GM-CSF antagonist	Bleomycin	Aggravation	Piguet *et al.* (1991c)
GM-CSF antagonist	Silicosis	Aggravation	Piguet *et al.* (1991c)
IL-1 antagonist	Bleomycin	Protection	P. F. Piguet (submitted, 1992)
IL-1 antagonist	Silicosis	Protection	P. F. Piguet (submitted, 1992)

[a] Antagonists are anticytokine antibodies, soluble receptor (TNF), or receptor antagonist (IL-1).

E. Induction of Fibrogenic Cytokines; Role of the Immune Response

In several types of pulmonary fibrosis, there are indications for an important role of the immune response, and particularly of T lymphocytes, in the expression of the fibrosis and in the production of fibrogenic cytokines. In the case of bleomycin-induced pulmonary fibrosis the following results were obtained: (1) Administration of bleomycin induced an influx of lymphocytes within the lung (Jones and Reeve, 1978). (2) Fibrotic reaction is markedly attenuated in athymic mice or in T lymphocyte-depleted mice (Schrier *et al.,* 1983; Piguet *et al.,* 1989); full expression of the fibrotic reaction requires T lymphocytes of both the CD4 and CD8 subsets, as indicated by *in vivo* depletion with monoclonal antibodies (Piguet *et al.,* 1989); depletion of T lymphocytes abrogates the TNF mRNA accumulation (Piguet *et al.,* 1989). (3) The MHC is involved in the expression of the susceptible/resistant phenotypes (Rossi *et al.,* 1987).

In the case of the pneumoconiosis, an involvement of the immune system is suggested by the following data: (1) An influx of T and B lymphocytes follows inhalation of particles (Kumar, 1989). (2) There is a less severe silicosis in athymic nude mice than in the euthymic nu/+ mice controls (Hubbard, 1989 and P. F. Piguet, unpublished observations), a difference that is, however, not as pronounced as with bleomycin. (3) There are various humoral (i.e., production of autoantibodies) manifestations (Doll, 1983). (4) There are particle-specific CD4 T lymphocytes present within the lungs (Saltini *et al.,* 1989). It is likely that the role and importance of the immune response in pneumoconiosis depend on the type of particles and host factors.

In interstitial lung diseases, an involvement of the immune system is mainly supported by the presence of T lymphocytes of both the CD4 and CD8 phenotype within the interstice.

F. Possibility of a Fibrogenic Cytokine Network

Several observations suggest that TNF might play a major role in pulmonary fibrosis (Piguet, 1990). Bleomycin- or silica-induced pulmonary fibrosis is associated with a marked and lasting increase of TNF mRNA within the lung; this can be prevented by anti-TNF antibody or by TNF inhibitors. An infusion of TNF can reproduce several of the findings observed during pulmonary fibrosis, such as alveolar damage, growth of fibroblasts, and collagen deposition. TNF might play a predominant role, either because it is produced in larger amounts than other fibrogenic cytokines, or because it is an inducer of other fibrogenic cytokines. More recent observations, however, show that IL-1 inhibitors (P. F. Piguet, unpublished observations) or anti-TGF-β antibodies (J. A. McDonald, personnal communication) can also markedly prevent experimental pulmonary fibrosis in mice; this suggests that the fibrogenic cytokines are part of a network, and that the blockade of one can disrupt the whole fibrogenic response.

III. OUTLOOK

The characterization of cytokines involved in fibrotic reactions is important, both for the understanding of the pathogenesis and for development of therapeutic treatment. Several fibrogenic cytokines have been fairly well characterized at the molecular and cell biology level, but their role in physiopathology, and particularly pulmonary fibrosis, is much less known and cannot be ascertained at this time. Information concerning cytokine production during the development of fibrosis is incomplete and the exploration of a cytokine role with inhibitors is just beginning.

Implications for therapy are of two sorts; first, it is evident that several of the drugs commonly used in the treatment of pulmonary fibrosis, such as steroids and cyclosporin, act by stopping (among others effects) cytokine, and particularly TNF, production. Second, the inhibition of experimental bleomycin-induced fibrosis or silicosis with infusions of interferon-γ or TNF inhibitors promises new opportunities for therapy.

Acknowledgments

This work has been performed with the collaboration of colleagues to whom I am indebted: Y. Kapanci, P. Vassalli, and G. Grau. I am also grateful to A. F. Rochat and C. Vesin for their technical collaboration. This work is supported by Swiss National Science foundation Grant No. 31-28855.90.

References

Antoniades, H. N., Bravo, M. A., Avila, R. E., *et al.* (1990). *J. Clin. Invest.* **86**, 1055–1064.

Bauman, M. D., Jetten, A. M., and Brody, A. R. (1987). *Chest* **91**, 15s–16s.

Beutler, B., and Cerami, A. (1988). *Biochemistry* **27**, 7575–7582.

Bissonnette, E., and Rolapleszczynski, M. (1989). *Inflammation* **13**, 329–339.

Bitterman, P. B., and Henke, C. A. (1991). *Chest* **99**, 81s–84s.

Bowden, D. H. (1987). *Exp. Lung Res.* **12**, 89–107.

Colby, T. V., and Churg, A. C. (1986). *Pathol. Annu.* **21**, 277–309.

D'Amore, P. A. (1990). *Cancer Metastasis Rev.* **9**, 227–238.

Dayer, J. M., Beutler, B., and Cerami, A. (1985). *J. Exp. Med.* **162**, 2163–2168.

Dinarello, C. A. (1989). *Adv. Immunol.* **44**, 153–204.

Doll, N. J. (1983). *Clin. Chest Med.* **4**, 3.

Fanslow, W. C., Sims, J. E., Sassenfeld, H., *et al.* (1990). *Science* **248**, 739–741.

Fuchs, H. J., Debs, R., Patton, J. S., and Liggit, H. D. (1990). *Diagn. Microbiol. Infect. Dis.* **13**, 397–404.

Goldring, S. R., Stephenson, M. L., Downie, E., Krane, S. M., and Korn, J. (1990). *J. Clin. Invest.* **85**, 798–803.

Hubbard, A. K. (1989). *Lab. Invest.* **61**, 46–52.

Hunninghake, G. W. (1984). *Am. Rev. Respir. Dis.* **129**, 569–572.

Hyde, D. M., Henderson, T. S., Giri, S. N., Tyler, N. K., and Stovall, M. Y. (1988). *Exp. Lung Res.* **14**, 687–704.

Jones, A. W., and Reeve, N. L. (1978). *J. Pathol.* **124**, 227–233.

Khalil, N., Bereznay, O., Sporn, M., and Greenberg, A. H. (1989). *J. Exp. Med.* **170**, 727–737.

Klagsbrun, M., and Edelman, E. R. (1989). *Arteriosclerosis* **9**, 269–278.

Kumar, R. K. (1989). *Am. J. Pathol.* **135**, 605–614.

Lassalle, P., Gosset, P., Aerts, C., *et al.* (1990). *Exp. Lung Res.* **16**, 73–80.

Lemaire, I. (1991). *Am. J. Pathol.* **138**, 487–495.

Lesslauer, W., Tabuchi, H., Gentz, R., *et al.* (1991). *Eur. J. Immunol.* **21**, 2883–2886.

Matsushima, K., Bano, M. J., Kidwell, W. R., and Oppenheim, J. J. (1985). *J. Immunol.* **134**, 904–909.

Mitchell, J., Woodcok-Mitchell, J., Reyolds, S., *et al.* (1989). *Lab. Invest.* **60**, 643–650.

Phipps, R. P., Baecher, C., Frelinger, J. G., Penney, D. P., Keng, P., and Brown, D. (1990). *Eur. J. Immunol.* **20**, 1723–1727.

Piguet, P. F. (1990). *Eur. Cytokine Network* **1**, 257–258.

Piguet, P. F. (1992). *In* "Xenobiotic Induced Inflammation: Roles of Cytokines and Growth Factors" (L. B. Schook and D. L. Laskin, eds). Academic Press, San Diego. In press.

Piguet, P. F., Collart, M. A., Grau, G. E., Kapanci, Y., and Vassalli, P. (1989). *J. Exp. Med.* **170**, 655–663.

Piguet, P. F., Collart, M. A., Grau, G. E., Sappino, A. P., and Vassalli, P. (1990a). *Nature (London)* **344**, 245–247.

Piguet, P. F., Grau, G. E., and Vassalli, P. (1990b). *Am. J. Pathol.* **136**, 103–110.

Piguet, P. F., Grau, G. E., and Vassalli, P. (1991a). *Immunol. Res.* **10**, 122–140.

Piguet, P. F., Grau, G. E., and de Kossodo, S. (1991c). Submitted.

Piguet, P. F., Chang, H. R., Tiberghien, P., and Hervé, P. (1992). *In* "The Clinical Applications of Cytokines: Role in Pathogenesis, Diagnosis and Therapy" (J. Oppenheim, ed.).

Postlethwaite, A. E., Lachman, L. B., Mainardi, C. L., and Kang, A. H. (1983). *J. Exp. Med.* **157**, 801–805.

Rifkin, D. B., and Moscatelli, D. (1989). *J. Cell Biol.* **109**, 1–6.

Roberts, A. B., and Sporn, M. B. (1989). *Am. Rev. Respir. Dis.* **140**, 1126–1128.

Roberts, A. B., Sporn, M. B., Assoian, R. K., *et al.* (1986). *Proc. Natl. Acad. Sci. U.S.A.* **83**, 4167–4171.

Rochemonteix-Galve, B., Dayer, J. M., and Junod, A. F. (1990). *Eur. Respir. J.* **3**, 653–664.

Rosenbloom, J., Feldman, G., Freundlich, B., and Jimenez, S. A. (1984). *Biochem. Biophys. Res. Commun.* **123**, 365–372.

Ross, R., Raines, E. W., and Bowen-Pope, D. F. (1986). *Cell* **46**, 155–169.

Rossi, G. A., Szapiel, S., Ferrans, V. J., and Crystal, R. G. (1987). *Am. Rev. Respir. Dis.* **135**, 448–455.

Saltini, C., Winestock, K., Kirby, M., Pinkston, P., and Crystal, R. G. (1989). *N. Engl. J. Med.* **320**, 1103–1109.

Sappino, A. P., Schurch, W., and Gabbiani, G. (1990). *Lab. Invest.* **63**, 144–161.

Schmidt, J. A., Mizel, S. B., Cohen, D., and Green, I. (1982). *J. Immunol.* **128**, 2177–2182.

Schrier, D. J., Phan, S. H., and McGary, M. (1983). *Am. Rev. Respir. Dis.* **127**, 614–617.

Spatafora, M., Merendino, A., Chiappara, G., *et al.* (1989). *Chest* **96**, 542–549.

Sprugel, K. H., McPherson, J. M., Clowes, A. W., and Ross, R. (1987). *Am. J. Pathol.* **129**, 601–613.

Sugarman, B. J., Aggarwal, B. B., Hass, P. E., Figari, I. S., Palladino, M. A., and Shepard, M. H. (1985). *Science* **230**, 943–945.

Suwabe, A., Takahashi, K., Yasui, S., Arai, S., and Sendo, F. (1988). *Am. J. Pathol.* **132,** 512–520.

Thornton, S. C., Por, S. B., Walsh, B. J., Penny, R., and Breit, S. N. (1990). *J. Leukocyte Biol.* **47,** 312–320.

Wahl, S. M., McCartney-Francis, N., and Mergenhagen, S. E. (1989). *Immunol. Today* **10,** 258–261.

Immune-Mediated Injury in Bacterial Meningitis

Karl Frei and Daniela Piani
Section of Clinical Immunology
Department of Neurosurgery
University Hospital
CH-8044 Zürich, Switzerland

Hans-Walter Pfister
Department of Neurology
University of Munich
Munich, Germany

Adriano Fontana
Section of Clinical Immunology
Department of Neurosurgery
University Hospital
CH-8044 Zürich, Switzerland

I. INTRODUCTION

Bacterial meningitis is a common disease worldwide. Since its historic description in 1805 as "epidemic cerebrospinal fever," physicians observed its almost uniformly fatal course until the introduction of antiserum in the early twentieth century (Flexner, 1913). Although the intrathecal administration of antiserum reduced the mortality of meningococcal meningitis from about 70 to 30%, the greatest decrease in mortality rates followed by the introduction of antibiotics (Colbrook and Kenny, 1936). However, bacterial meningitis continues to be an important cause of morbidity and morality despite the introduction of and continued improvement in antibiotics and despite the progress made on management with fluids of endotoxic shock and vascular

International Review of Experimental Pathology, Volume 34B

failure (Dodge, 1986; Smith, 1988). Case fatality rates for the three most common etiologic agents of bacteria meningitis, *Haemophilus influenzae, Neisseria meningitidis,* and *Streptococcus pneumoniae,* were 6, 10, and 25%, respectively, in the United States from 1978 to 1981. These mortality rates have changed little over the past 30 years. In addition, there is a high incidence of long-term neurologic sequelae in children and adults with bacterial meningitis (Bohr *et al.,* 1984; Pomeroy *et al.,* 1990). Early diagnosis of these cases is one of the key elements that determines the outcome of the patient. Cultures of blood and cerebrospinal fluid (CSF) for detection of the etiologic agent have the drawback of the time required for cultures to become "positive." In addition, measurements of cell counts and concentrations of protein and glucose in the CSF may not always be absolutely diagnostic, as the ranges of the data in bacterial meningitis overlap significantly with those in viral meningitis (Weinstein, 1985; Bolan and Barza, 1985). There is increasing evidence that cytokines, in addition to their essential role in the periphery during bacterial and viral infections, mediate many host responses in infectious diseases of the central nervous system (CNS).

II. TNF-α: A KEY MEDIATOR IN BACTERIAL MENINGITIS

A number of experimental findings support the role of interleukin-1 (IL-1) and tumor necrosis factor-α (TNF-α) as key mediators of host responses to microbial invasion and immunological insults. When passively immunized with antisera against TNF-α, mice were found to be protected against the lethal effect of endotoxin (Beutler *et al.,* 1985). Furthermore, intravenous infusion of TNF-α into rats causes a hemorrhagic necrosis that is indistinguishable from the pathologic effects seen after endotoxin administration (Tracey *et al.,* 1986).

In bacterial meningitis major pathological findings are characterized by (1) extensive infiltration of the leptomeninges and perivascular spaces with leukocytes and (2) cerebrospinal fluid changes, including polymorphonuclear pleocytosis, increased protein, and intracranial hypertension. In the pathophysiology of bacterial meningitis, leukocyte-derived factors such as polyunsaturated fatty acids and reactive oxygen intermediates as well as the production of cytokines in the nervous system may be decisive (for review see Tunkel and Scheld, 1991). To provide evidence for a pathogenetic role of cytokines—especially TNF-α—in bacterial meningitis, the presence of TNF-α and various interleukins and colony-stimulating factors were assessed in the CSF in an experimental animal model as well as in patients with meningitis. After intracerebral, but not systemic, infection with *Listeria monocytogenes* in mice, TNF-α was detected in the CSF as early as 3 hr after infection (100 to 200 U/ml), reaching maximal levels after 48 hr (up to

16,000 U/ml). In contrast, TNF-α was not found in the CSF of mice suffering from severe lymphocytic choriomeningitis induced by intracerebral infection with lymphocytic choriomeningitis virus (LCMV) (Leist *et al.,* 1988). This difference is striking in that both model infections led to massive infiltration of polymorphonuclear and mononuclear leukocytes into the meninges and CSF. Analogously, TNF-α was only detected in the CSF of patients with bacterial but not viral meningitis (Fig. 1) (Leist *et al.,* 1988; Nadal *et al.,* 1989). In contrast to CSF, the serum of patients with bacterial meningitis contained no or only small amounts of TNF-α (Leist *et al.,* 1988; Nadal *et al.,* 1989). These data were reproduced in a number of studies. TNF-α concentrations in the CSF were found to correlate with CSF protein and endotoxin concentrations, bacterial density, and outcome of disease

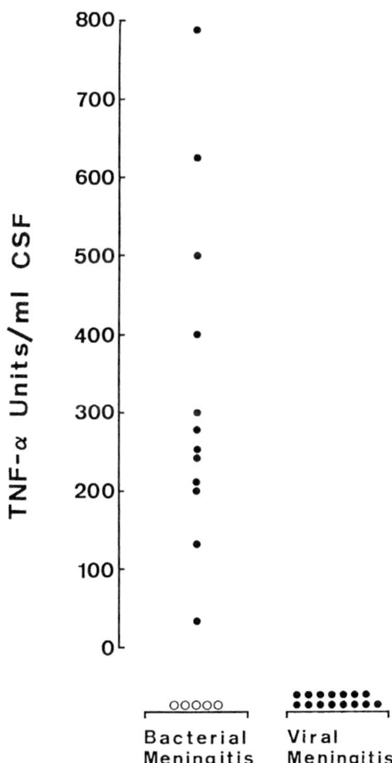

Fig. 1. Presence of TNF-α in CSF of patients with acute bacterial meningitis but not viral meningitis. TNF-α was quantitated in the CSF of 17 patients with bacterial meningitis and of 15 patients with viral meningitis. The CSF was collected within 48 hr after admission of the patients to the hospital. In five patients (o) with bacterial meningitis, the CSF samples were taken later in the course of disease, on days 3 to 9. TNF-α was measured using a previously described cytotoxic assay (Frei *et al.,* 1987).

(Arditi *et al.,* 1990), as well as with the amount of IL-1β (Mustafa *et al.,* 1989). In infants with bacterial meningitis, a significantly higher percentage of children who died had IL-1 CSF concentrations above 500 pg/ml when compared with infants who survived. No such correlation was found for TNF-α (McCracken *et al.,* 1989). At the time of diagnosis, IL-1β was detected also in TNF-α-negative CSF samples from patients with viral meningitis (Ramilo *et al.,* 1990). Besides TNF-α and IL-1, the CSF of patients with bacterial meningitis also contained macrophage colony-stimulating factor (M-CSF) and granulocyte colony-stimulating factor (G-CSF) (Table I), which may contribute to the activation of infiltrating monocytes and granulocytes, respectively (Gallo *et al.,* 1990; Frei *et al.,* 1991; Shimoda *et al.,* 1991).

Injection of meningococcal lipopolysaccharide (LPS) into the subarachnoid space of rabbits induced the sequential appearance of TNF-α, IL-1, and IL-6 followed by migration of leukocytes into the CSF compartment (Waage *et al.,* 1989). Whereas injection of LPS into the subarachnoidal space did not lead to the appearance of circulating TNF-α, systemic endotoxinemia was paralleled by TNF-α only in the blood, and not in the CSF (Waage *et al.,* 1989). Furthermore, TNF-α, IL-1α, macrophage inflammatory protein-1 (MIP-1) and MIP-2 injected intracisternally into rabbits induced enhanced blood–brain barrier permeability, leukocytosis in CSF, and brain edema (Saukkonen *et al.,* 1990; Ramilo *et al.,* 1990). After intracisternal infection

Table I. Intrathecal Synthesis of Cytokines in Infectious Meningitis

	Cerebrospinal fluid	
Disease	Positive	Negative
Bacterial meningitis	TNF-α	IFN-γ
	IL-1β	
	IL-3	
	IL-6	
	IL-8	
	M-CSF	
	G-CSF	
	GM-CSF	
	L-TGF-β	
Viral meningitis/encephalitis	IFN-γ	TNF-α
	IL-1β	IL-2
	IL-6	IL-3
	IL-8	IL-4
	M-CSF	IL-5
	GM-CSF	
	L-TGF-β	

with heat-killed *Streptococcus pneumoniae,* antibodies to TNF-α or to IL-1 prevented CSF leukocytosis whereas anti-MIP-1 and anti-MIP-2 antibodies were ineffective. Though all antibodies reduced the CSF protein concentration, only antibody to TNF-α was also protective against brain edema (Saukkonen *et al.,* 1990). The same data were observed when investigating antibodies to both IL-1β and TNF-α in rabbits injected with *H. influenzae* type b lipooligosaccharide (Ramilo *et al.,* 1990).

III. TGF-β: EFFECT IN PNEUMOCOCCAL MENINGITIS

In bacterial meningitis, macrophages and granulocytes seem to play a key role. Dexamethasone, indomethacin, and superoxide dismutase have been shown to attenuate the development of microvascular changes during the early phase of experimental meningitis (Pfister *et al.,* 1990). These data point to an involvement of molecules from the arachidonic acid metabolism and of reactive oxygen intermediates. Clinical trials with dexamethasone provide evidence of a beneficial effect of antiinflammatory therapy in infants and children with bacterial meningitis (Odio *et al.,* 1991).

Because TGF-β leads to macrophage deactivation (Tsunawaki *et al.,* 1988), to inhibition of production of cytokines such as TNF-α (Espevik *et al.,* 1987), and to decreased endothelial granulocyte adhesion (Gamble and Vadas, 1988), we investigated whether TGF-β might influence regional cerebral blood flow (rCBF), intracranial pressure (ICP), and brain edema formation during the early phase of experimental meningitis. In a well-characterized meningitis model (Pfister *et al.,* 1990), rats were inoculated intracisternally (i.c.) with live pneumococci and were found to develop a severe meningitis within 6–12 hr (Fig. 2). As early as within the first 4 hr after i.c. challenge with live pneumococci, an increase of rCBF and ICP can be monitored. A single intraperitoneal (i.p.) injection of rHu-TGF-β2 (10 μg) 1 hr before bacterial infection prevented the changes in rCBF, ICP, and brain water content (Pfister *et al.,* 1992). The beneficial effects of TGF-β on the initial phase following pneumococcal inocculation seems to be TNF-α independent because (1) i.c. or i.p. injections of neutralizing anti-TNF-α antibodies did not signficantly influence rCBF, ICP, and brain edema and (2) TNF-α was only occasionally detected at low levels in CSF at 4 hr after pneumococcal infection. However, at later time points, e.g., at 6 hr after bacterial inoculation, TNF-α can be detected in CSF and anti-TNF-α antibodies reduced pleocytosis. Thus, in contrast to the initial phase of bacterial meningitis, TNF-α is crucially involved in the pathogenesis of meningitis at later stages. In our model, neither the definite site of action of TGF-β nor the mechanisms underlying the beneficial effect of TGF-β on the cerebrovavular changes are known.

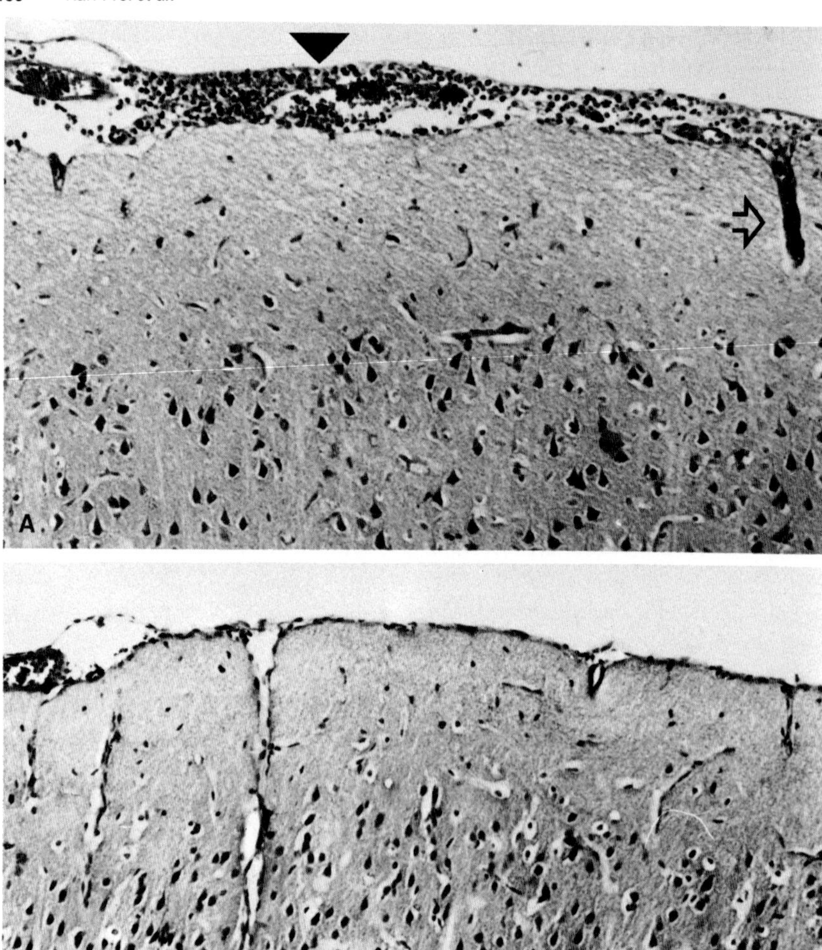

Fig. 2. Micrographs of brain sections of rats after intracisternal injection of viable pneumococcus (a) or phosphate-buffered saline (PBS) (b). (a) Parietal brain cortex, 12 hr after i.c. injection of pneumococcus (75 μl, 10^7 CFU/ml): acute meningitis with polymorphonuclear leukocytes and some mononuclear cells in the enlarged leptomeningeal space (solid arrow), located predominantly perivenous, extending along blood vessels into the uppermost layer of the cortex (open arrow). Giemsa stain ($\times$140). (b) Control parietal brain cortex, 12 hr after i.c. injection of PBS (75 μl): no meningeal infiltration. Hematoxylin and eosin ($\times$140).

IV. NEURONAL CELL DEATH IN BACTERIAL MENINGITIS

In bacterial meningitis, the pathogenesis of major neurological sequelae, including mental retardation, seizures, deafness, and hemiparesis, is only poorly understood. In a recent prospective study of 185 infants and children with acute bacterial meningitis, 1 month after onset of disease, 69 children (37%) were found to have neurologic abnormalities (Pomeroy *et al.,* 1990). Encephalopathy with death of neuronal cells has generally been thought to result from inflammation, brain edema, occlusion of meningeal vessels, and interference with cerebral metabolism by invading microorganisms and their toxins.

Macrophages taken from mycobacteria (BCG)-infected mice or activated by bacterial LPS destroy tumor cells in tissue culture through the production of hydrogen peroxide, proteases, and TNF-α (Old, 1985; Beutler and Cerami, 1986). However, tumor cell selectivity is not absolute. Examples of TNF-α-mediated cytotoxicity exerted on nontransformed cells are oligodendrocytes (Robbins *et al.,* 1987) in the brain and insulin-producing pancreatic β islet cells (Campbell *et al.,* 1988). Though there is clear evidence for an involvement of TNF-α and other cytokines in the development of meningeal inflammation, the contribution of cytokines to facilitate irreversible neuronal injury has not been assessed so far. In a recent study we demonstrated that neither TNF-α nor IL-1β, IL-6, IFN-α/β, or IFN-γ induce morphological changes in cultured cerebellar neurons. Despite of the presence of the respective cytokines, neurons remained adherent and connected to each other through neuronal processes (Piani *et al.,* 1992). Only the combined treatment of neurons with high doses of TNF-α (1000 U/ml) and IL-1β (10 ng/ml) caused moderate cytotoxicity (20%) as measured by the colorimetric MTT (tetrazolium) assay. When investigating the effect of hydrogen peroxide, the reaction product of superoxide, it was found that hydrogen peroxide induces extensive neuronal damage (Piani *et al.,* 1991b). The neurotoxic effect is of note because superoxide and hydrogen peroxide have been shown to be secreted by TNF-α-stimulated macrophages, including brain microglial cells, or by leukocytes (Colton and Gilbert, 1987; Sonderer *et al.,* 1987). However, macrophage-induced neurotoxicity as observed in coculture experiments can only partially be prevented by superoxide dismutase and catalase. Recently, macrophages were found to secrete excitatory amino acids (glutamate), which potentially kills N-methyl-D-aspartate (NMDA) receptor-positive neurons in culture (Fig. 3) (Piani *et al.,* 1991). Thus, in bacterial meningitis, the neurologic sequelae being observed in severely diseased patients may be due to inappropriate release of cytokines, of reactive oxygen intermediates, and of L-glutamate secreted by inflammatory cells invading the CNS. Treatment of bacterial meningitis should in the future comprise not only bactericidal antibiotics,

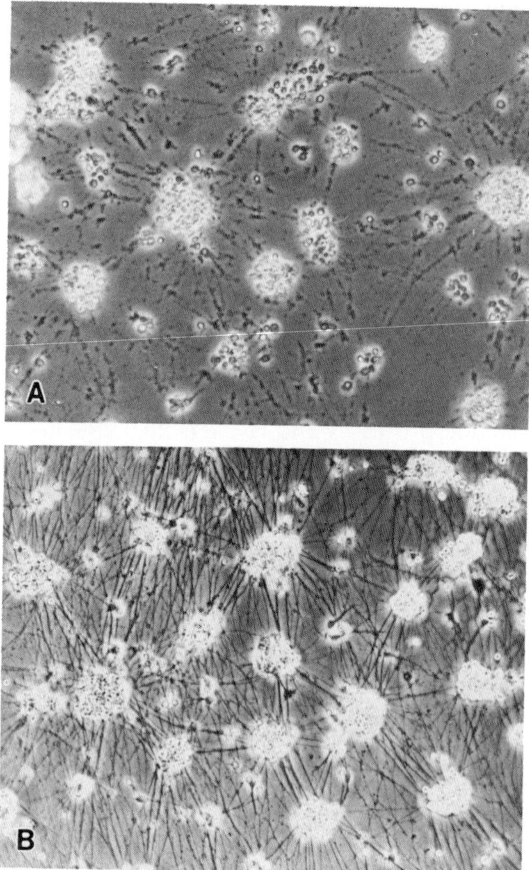

Fig. 3. Microglial cells secrete neurotoxic molecules. Cerebellar neurons, grown for 5 days on laminin-coated coverslips, were either exposed to (a) supernatant of microglial cells (2.5%, v/v) or to (b) media control; 24 hr later, phase-contrast photomicrographs were taken (×125).

but also compounds that block the production and/or effects of mediators of inflammation.

V. SUMMARY

Cytokines are involved in the host response to bacterial infections. In bacterial meningitis, intrathecal synthesis of TNF-α and IL-1 is likely to contribute to CNS injury by recruitment and activation of inflammatory cells with subsequent release of toxic factors, such as reactive oxygen intermediates and excitatory amino acids (glutamate), leading to neuronal cell death with neurologic sequelae. In rats with experimental meningitis, pretreatment with TGF-β inhibits cerebrovascular changes and brain edema formation in the early, TNF-α-independent phase. Provided its local production in bacterial infection, TGF-β may comprise a host factor interfering with immune pathologic events altering the integrity of the endothelial barrier.

Acknowledgments

This work has been supported by the Swiss National Science Foundation (Project No. 31-28402.90), Sandoz Ltd., Basel, Switzerland, and the Deutsche Forschungsgemeinschaft (Project No. 24613-1).

References

Arditi, M., Manogue, K. R., Caplan, M., and Yogev, R. (1990). *J. Infect. Dis.* **162**, 139.

Beutler, B., and Cerami, A. (1986). *Nature (London)* **320**, 584.

Beutler, B., Milsark, I. W., and Cerami, A. (1985). *Science* **229**, 869.

Bohr, V., Paulson, O., and Rasmussen, N. (1984). *Arch. Neurol.* **41**, 1045.

Bolan, G., and Barza, M. (1985). *Med. Clin. N. Am.* **69**, 231.

Campbell, I. L., Isarco, A., and Harrison, L. C. (1988). *J. Immunol.* **141**, 2325.

Colbrook, L., and Kenny, M. (1946). *Lancet* **i**, 1279.

Colton, C. A., and Gilbert, D. L. (1987). *FEBS Lett.* **223**, 284.

Dodge, P. R. (1986). *Pediatr. Infect. Dis. J.* **5**, 618.

Espevik, T., Figari, I. S., Shalaby, M. R., Lackides, G. A., Lewis, G. D., Shepard, H. M., and Palladino, M. (1987). *J. Exp. Med.* **166**, 571.

Flexner, S. (1913). *J. Exp. Med.* **17**, 553.

Frei, K., Siepl, C., Groscurth, P., Bodmer, S., Schwerdel, C., and Fontana, A. (1987). *Eur. J. Immunol.* **17**, 1271.

Frei, K., Leist, T. P., Meager, A., Gallo, P., Leppert, D., Zinkernagel, R. M., and Fontana, A. (1988). *J. Exp. Med.* **168**, 449.

Frei, K., Nadal, D., and Fontana, A. (1990). *Ann. N.Y. Acad. Sci.* **594**, 326.

Frei, K., Nadal, D., Ralph, P., and Fontana, A. (1991). *In* "Cellular and Cytokine Networks in Tissue Immunity" (M. Meltzer and A. Mantovani, eds.), pp. 91–98. Wiley-Liss, New York.

Gallo, P., Pagni, S., Giometto, B., Piccinno, M. G., Bozza, F., Argentiero, V., and Tavolato, B. (1990). *J. Neuroimmunol.* **29**, 105.

Gamble, J. R., and Vadas, M. A. (1988). *Science* **242**, 97.

Leist, T. P., Frei, K., Kam-Hansen, S., Zinkernagel, R. M., and Fontana, A. (1988). *J. Exp. Med.* **167**, 1743.

McCracken, G. H., Mustafa, M. M., Ramilo, O., Olsen, K. D., and Risser, R. C. (1989). *Pediatr. Infect. Dis. J.* **8**, 155.

Mustafa, M., Lebel, M. H., Ramilo, O., Olsen, K. D., Reisch, J. S., Beutler, B., and McCracken, G. H., Jr. (1989). *J. Pediatr.* **115**, 208.

Nadal, D., Leppert, D., Frei, K., Gallo, P., Lamche, H., and Fontana, A. (1989). *Arch. Dis. Child.* **64**, 1274.

Odio, C. M., Faingezicht, I., Paris, M., Nassar, M., Baltodano, A., Roger, J., Saez-Llorens, X., Olsen, K. D., and McCracken, G.H. (1991). *N. Engl. J. Med.* **324**, 1525.

Old, L. J. (1985). *Science* **230**, 630.

Pfister, H. W., Koedel, U., Haberl, R. L., Dirnagl, U., Feiden, W., Ruckdeschel, G., and Einhäupl, K. M. (1990). *J. Cereb. Blood Flow Metab.* **10**, 914.

Pfister, H. W., Frei, K., Ottnad, B., Koedel, U., Tomasz, A., and Fontana, A. (1992). *J. Exp. Med.* **176**, 265.

Piani, D., Frei, K., Do, K. Q., Cuénod, M., and Fontana, A. (1991). *Neurosci. Lett.* **133**, 159.

Piani, D., Spranger, M., Frei, K., Schaffner, A., and Fontana, A. (1992). *Eur. J. Immunol.* **22**, 2429.

Pomeroy, S. L., Homes, S. J., Dodge, P. R., and Feigin, R. D. (1990). *N. Engl. J. Med.* **323**, 1651.

Ramilo, O., Mustafa, M. M., Porter, J., Saez-Llorens, X., Mertsola, J., Olson, K. D., Luby, J. P., Beutler, B., and McCracken, G. H. (1990). *Am. J. Dis. Child.* **144**, 349.

Robbins, D. S., Shirazi, Y., Drysdale, B.-E., Lieberman, A., Shin, H. S., and Shin, M. L. (1987). *J. Immunol.* **139**, 2593.

Saukkonen, K., Sande, S., Cioffe, C., Wolpe, S., Sherry, B., Cerami, A., and Tuomanen, E. (1990). *J. Exp. Med.* **171**, 439.

Shimoda, K., Okamura, S., Omori, F., Mizuno, Y., Hara, T., Aoki, T., Ueda, K., and Niho, Y. (1991). *Blood* **77**, 2214.

Smith, A. L. (1988). *N. Engl. J. Med.* **319**, 1012.

Sonderer, B., Wild, P., Wyler, R., Fontana, A., Peterhans, E., and Schwyzer, M. (1987). *J. Leukocyte Biol.* **42**, 463.

Tracey, K. J., Beutler, B., Lowry, S. F., Merryweather, J., Wolpe, S., Milsark, I. W., Hairi, R. J., Fahey, T. J., III, Zentella, A., Albert, J. D., Shires, G. T., and Cerami, A. (1986). *Science* **234**, 47.

Tsunawaki, S., Sporn, M., Ding, A., and Nathan, C. (1988). *Nature (London)* **334**, 260.

Tunkel, A. R., and Scheld, W. M. (1991). *In* "Infections of the Central Nervous System" (H. P. Lambert, ed.), pp. 1–15. B. C. Decker, Philadelphia.

Waage, A., Halstensen, A., Shalaby, R., Brandtzaeg, P., Kirulf, P., and Espevik, T. (1989). *J. Exp. Med.* **170**, 1859.

Weinstein, L. (1985). *Med. Clin. N. Am.* **69**, 219.

Clinical Experiences with Interferon-α and Interferon-γ

Gerhard G. Steinmann
Clinical Research
Boehringer Ingelheim
D-7950 Biberach, Germany

Frank Rosenkaimer and Gerhard Leitz
Corporate Medicine
Boehringer Ingelheim
Ingelheim, Germany

I. THE INTERFERON FAMILY

Interferon was initially identified by Isaacs and Lindenmann (1957) as a soluble factor that inhibited infection of chick chorioallantoic membranes by influenza A virus. Since the discovery and naming of interferon, a whole family of naturally occurring proteins has been detected sharing antiviral, immunomodulatory, and antiproliferative properties. In addition, interferons are potent regulators of cell gene expression, structure, and function. Interferons, in particular recombinant interferon-α, possess considerable direct antiproliferative activities and are attractive anticancer agents (Strander, 1986). Their antiproliferative effects have been the most thoroughly studied activity of all biological response modifiers, whereas recombinant interferon-γ exerts immunomodulatory effects not seen with other interferons (Jaffe and Sherwin, 1986).

Interferons can be subdivided into two classes according to their acid stability. The first class, which is acid proof, consists of three families, i.e., α, β, and ω. The second class consists of interferon-γ, which is not acid proof

Table I. Classification of Human Interferons

Characteristic	Interferon class			
	IFN-α	IFN-β	IFN-ω	IFN-γ
Natural source	Leukocytes, fibroblasts	Fibroblasts, leukocytes	Leukocytes	T lymphocytes
Number of species	14	1	1	1
Introns	−	−	−	+
Chromosomal location (human)	9, short arm	9, short arm	9, short arm	12, long arm T
Inducers	Viruses, bacteria, poly(I:C)	Viruses, bacteria, poly(I:C)	Viruses	mitogens, specific antigens
Molecular mass (kDa)	19	22	24	45 (dimer)

(see Table I). Interferon-α is predominantly produced by leukocytes, B cells, T cells, null cells, and macrophages following exposure to B cell mitogens, viruses, foreign cells, or tumor cells. Interferon-β is predominantly produced by fibroblasts following exposure to viruses or foreign nucleic acids. Interferon-ω is produced by lymphocytes after exposure to viruses, and interferon-γ is produced by T lymphocytes following stimulation with T cell mitogens, specific antigens, or interleukin-2.

There are at least 18 interferon-α genes (including pseudogenes), one interferon-β gene, and one interferon-γ gene. Interferon-α and interferon-β have approximately 45% homology at the nucleic acid level; interferon-γ shares essentially no similarities with the other interferons. A fourth family of genes with an approximate deviation in coding sequence from interferon-α and interferon-β of 30 and 50%, respectively, has recently been designated interferon-ω.

The interferon-α, -β, and -ω genes are located at chromosome 9p21-p22. The interferon-γ gene is found on chromosome 12q24.1. The nucleotide sequences for the interferon-α, -β, and -γ genes have been extensively described, and the amino acid sequences of the gene products are known (Goeddel *et al.*, 1981; Streuli *et al.*, 1980). The interferon-α genes encode proteins of approximately 165 or 166 amino acids.

Interferon-α-2c is a member of the human interferon-α family of proteins (Dworkin-Rastl *et al.*, 1982, 1983). It is produced by an *Escherichia coli* strain carrying the recombinant plasmid with a cDNA, originally isolated from a Sendai virus-induced human cell line (Namalwa).

Only a single interferon-β gene, also encoding a protein of 165 amino acids, has so far been identified, and there appears to be a single interferon-γ gene encoding a protein of 143 amino acids (Trent *et al.*, 1982). Interferon-γ-1b is manufactured by a gene encoding for the naturally occurring amino acid sequence and consists of noncovalent dimers. Finally, a single functional ω gene encodes 172 amino acids.

II. PHARMACOLOGY AND MODE OF ACTION OF INTERFERONS

The use of interferon-α in the treatment of malignant hematological diseases and solid tumors is now well established in clinical practice. However, the exact mechanism of action still remains to be described. This lack of understanding is severe handicap in directing interferons to more therapeutic success.

Results from pharmacological studies have shown that interferon-α is pharmacodynamically active in terms of at least four different biological dimensions: (1) antiviral effects, (2) antiproliferative effects, (3) differentiation-inducing effects, and (4) immunomodulatory effects (see Table II).

Interferon-α-2c has, like other recombinant interferon-α family members,

Table II. Mode of Action of Interferon-α

Antiviral effects
    2′,5′-Oligoadenylate synthetase (+)
    Mx protein (+)

Direct antiproliferative effects
    Growth cycle arrest (+)
    Prevention of DNA sequence alteration (+)
    B cell growth factor response of hairy cells (−)

Differentiation-inducing effects
    Protein kinases (+)
    Oncogen expression (+)
    Cyclic nucleotides and prostaglandins (+)
    Surface antigen expression (+)
    Surface microviscosity (+)

Immunomodulatory effects
    Natural killer activity (+)
    Macrophage tumoricidal activity (+)
    Antibody-dependent cellular cytotoxicity (+)
    Fc receptor expression (+)
    Antibody production (IgG+/IgM−)

displayed antiviral activity against a variety of viruses *in vitro* and *in vivo*. Using bovine kidney cells as the target, influenza virus strains Ao/WSN, fowl plague, B-Lee, and the paramyxovirus Newcastle disease virus were highly sensitive to interferon-α-2c. In an African green monkey model for herpes simplex virus infection of the cornea, topical administration of low-dose interferon-α-2c resulted in reduced severity of keratitis. In combination with a low (and per se ineffective) dose of interferon-γ, interferon-α-2c partially prevented viral infections and subsequent development of keratitis.

From clinical trials with patients suffering from herpes of the cornea, we know that the results of the preclinical herpes studies have been highly predictive for human therapy. Additionally, interferon-α-2c significantly reduced healing time in clinical trials in combination with chemotherapeutic agents (e.g., trifluorothymidine or acyclovir). Therefore, the assessment of antiviral activities of interferon-α-2c by *in vitro* and *in vivo* models was a valid predictor for the clinical efficacy in viral diseases. Because animal models of chronic myelogenous leukemia (CML) have pointed at a viral genesis (Tanaka and Craig, 1970; DePaoli *et al.,* 1973), the antiviral activity of interferon-α might play a role in clinical therapy of CML as well.

With regard to antiproliferative activities of interferon-α observed in a variety of animal tumor models, evidence for both the direct effects on the tumor cells and indirect effects on the immune system of the host have been substantiated. In particular, animal models with large volume disease demonstrated activity. Animal models for hairy cell leukemia, however, are not available to date. Several studies have demonstrated that the proliferation of human hairy cells cultured *in vitro* in the presence of B cell growth factor is inhibited (Paganelli *et al.,* 1986; Sigaux *et al.,* 1987; Genot *et al.,* 1987) and that the phenotype of hairy cells is modulated (Fattorossi *et al.,* 1987). Similarly, interferon-α has been shown to suppress the growth of colonies of granulocytes and monocytes from normal donors and from patients with CML (Verma *et al.,* 1978; Neuman and Fauser, 1982; Oladipupo-Williams *et al.,* 1981). Interferon-α-2c inhibited to varying extents the proliferation of a variety of human tumor cell lines *in vitro.* Tumor cell types sensitive to the growth-inhibiting activity of the interferon-α-2c include carcinomas of the larynx, lung, breast, colon, and lymphoma cells. In clonogenic growth assays of primary tumor cells, colony formation of cells derived from a number of pancreatic, gastric, and colon cancer specimens was inhibited; the majority of tumors, however, were resistant. In a mouse tumor model, interferon-α-2c inhibited growth of two out of five human osteosarcoma xenotransplants in immunodeficient nude mice.

The interferon-α family members often simultaneously promote the differentiation of normal and tumor cell types (Chen and Najor, 1987) and may have an autoregulatory role, because some cell lines produce interferon-α

during the phase of terminal differentiation. Such cell lines increase their levels of 2′,5′-oligoadenylate synthetase in S phase and decrease them in the G_2 phase.

Analyses of immunomodulatory effects of the interferon-α family by *in vivo* models is difficult due to the species restriction of most of the biological effects. Human studies result in more reliable data. Treatment with human interferon-α-2c increased the expression of class II major histocompatibility complex antigens on splenic hairy cells isolated from patients with hairy cell leukemia. In contrast, interferon-α-2c had no effect on the expression of these antigens in breast carcinoma cells. Interferon-α-2c induced expression of the gene encoding tumor necrosis factor in a human promyelocytic leukemia cell line, but had no effect on the oxidative response of primary human polymorphonuclear leukocytes. In a phase I clinical trial of low-dose interferon-α-2c (6 μg per day, intramuscular application), natural killer cell activity of isolated peripheral blood lymphocytes was enhanced in 7 out of 10 patients. In two additional patients a transient increase was observed, whereas in one other patient a decrease of natural cytotoxicity was found (Nerl *et al.,* 1989).

Interferon-γ possesses a wide range of immunomodulatory activities, indicating potential clinical efficacy against infectious and inflammatory diseases. The extensive data that have accumulated in the scientific literature since recombinant interferon-γ (rIFN-γ) from various species has become available identify rIFN-γ as the predominant phagocyte-activating factor and enhancer of cell-mediated responses (Nathan *et al.,* 1983). There have been numerous *in vivo* studies to evaluate the effect of interferon-γ-1b in animals infected with viruses, bacteria, or parasites. The results of most of these studies demonstrate that interferon-γ-1b exerts potent antimicrobial activity *in vivo* when administered as a single agent. Additionally, enhanced activity is observed against specific infections (*Toxoplasma gondii, Leishmania donovani, Staphylococcus aureus, Listeria monocytogenes*), when interferon-γ-1b is used in combination treatments with other cytokines or antimicrobial agents. The potential to inhibit viral infections was assessed by examining Bolivian squirrel monkeys infected with encephalomyocarditis virus and African green monkeys infected with simian varicella virus, foamy virus, and Epstein–Barr-like herpes virus, and herpes simplex virus. Protection against sporozoite but not trophozoite infection examined in studies of malaria infection of rhesus monkeys was observed as a dose-dependent effect of the treatment with interferon-γ-1b (Buchmeier and Schreiber, 1985; Kiderlen *et al.,* 1984; McCabe *et al.,* 1984; Murray *et al.,* 1983).

Additional *in vivo* studies demonstrated that interferon-γ-1b is able (1) to enhance the antibody response to specific antigens, suggesting a potential use as a vaccine adjuvant, (2) to increase the incidence and severity of collagen-induced arthritis, and (3) to protect animals from lethal doses of irradiation.

III. CLINICAL EFFICACY OF INTERFERONS

It has only been a decade since recombinant interferons could be provided for preclinical and clinical research. The exuberant enthusiasm of the late 1970s and early 1980s, however, was followed by disillusion. By no means did interferons turn out to be wonder drugs, the "body's own substances to treat cancer and virus infections without side effects." Interferons have nevertheless found their place in therapy of several malignant and viral diseases. Table III lists the current marketing registrations of interferon-α for oncological indications.

Most impressive is the effect of interferon-α in hairy cell leukemia, with a remission rate of approximately 85% (see Table IV). It was proved that recombinant interferon-α is active against bulky diseases. Counts of neutrophils, granulocytes, and thrombocytes, as well as hemoglobin values, increase noticeably under the interferon therapy. Survival is prolonged because lethal complications (i.e., severe infections and blood loss) can be prevented. Although the duration of remissions usually exceeds 2 years,

Table III. Worldwide Registration of Interferon-α in Oncological Indications

Type of cancer	Number of countries
Hairy cell leukemia	45
Kaposi's sarcoma	36
Plasmocytoma	28
Malignant melanoma	27
Chronic myelogenous leukemia	18
Non-Hodgkin's lymphoma	10
Chronic lymphocytic leukemia, cutaneous T cell lymphoma, mycosis fungoides	
Renal cell carcinoma	9
Transitional cell carcinoma	1
Ovarian carcinoma	1
Basal cell carcinoma	1
Glioblastoma	1
Advanced cancer	1

Table IV. Interferon-α in the Treatment of Malignancies

Malignancy	Response rates[a]
Leukemias/lymphomas	
Hairy cell leukemia	85%
Chronic myelogenous leukemia, chronic phase	66%
Cutaneous T cell lymphoma	65%
Macroglobulinemia	51%
Non-Hodgkin's lymphoma	
Low-grade malignancy	37%
High-grade malignancy	14%
Plasmocytoma (IgA, light chain)	27%
Solid tumors	
Basal cell carcinoma	86%
Carcinoid	43%
Advanced renal cell carcinoma	41%
Kaposi's sarcoma	35%
Ovarian carcinoma	19%
Advanced malignant melanoma	15%
Breast carcinoma	7%
Colorectal carcinoma	3%

[a] Response rates in terms of complete plus partial remission.

leukemic cells are not totally eliminated. The rate of complete remissions seems to be lower than anticipated. Usually, interferon-α is only able to balance the malignant growth and to keep the leukemic cells in check. The efficacy of interferon-α is strong enough to prevent death caused by hairy cell leukemia, but continuous therapy is necessary.

A second achievement was the treatment of chronic myelogenous leukemia (Table IV). Up to 80% of the patients experienced an improvement in terms of leukocytosis, anemia, and splenomegaly. Very often (40%) patients achieve normal metaphases in the bone marrow. In 15% of the patients the Philadelphia chromosome disappears.

Another high success rate was observed in thrombocytosis, a condition associated with multiple myeloproliferative diseases, including polycythemia rubra vera. Interferon-α is also effective against T cell lymphoma, nodular non-Hodgkin's lymphoma, macroglobulinemia, and multiple myeloma producing IgA and light chains (Table IV).

Intralesional application of interferons in basal cell carcinoma proved to be successful (86% complete responses). Of the patients, 81% were free of tumor 1 year after treatment. Kaposi's sarcoma was one of the first diseases to show promising remission rates. Nevertheless, even high doses seem to induce regressions only in 35% of patients. Other tumors with sensitivity to interferons include pulmonary hemangiomatosis, lymphangioma, renal cell carcinoma, malignant melanoma, and ovarian carcinoma. Neuroendocrine tumors also turned out to be treatable by interferon-α: carcinoids responded in 43% of the cases to treatment (Oberg, 1988). Interferon-α also exhibited substantial activity in virus-induced lesions. These disease states include juvenile laryngeal papillomatosis, condylomata accuminata, and HPV-infections of the cervical mucosa. Viral hepatitis (B and non-A/non-B) are now also established indications for interferon-α treatment.

Recently, the clinical efficacy of interferon-γ-1b in reducing the frequency and severity of serious infections in patients with chronic granulomatous disease (CGD) was described (International Chronic Granulomatous Disease Cooperative Study Group, 1991). CGD is an inherited disorder in which phagocytes ingest but do not kill catalase-positive microorganisms, because the cells fail to generate oxygen metabolites that normally kill these microbes. CGD patients suffer from recurrent pyogenic and fungal infections and granulomatous lesions, which often require extended periods of hospitalization with parenteral antibiotic therapy. Morbidity and mortality of patients with CGD is distressingly high (Curnutte *et al.*, 1988).

In two pilot studies interferon-γ-1b was able to correct the deficient phagocyte activity in CGD patients. A worldwide phase III study (randomized, double blind, placebo controlled) provided convincing evidence that interferon-γ-1b (50 μg/m^2, three times per week, s.c.) can significantly reduce the frequency and severity of serious infections in CGD patients. Interferon-γ-1b reduced the relative risk of serious infections by ~70% compared to placebo and reduced the length of hospitalization by one-third (International Chronic Granulomatous Disease Cooperative Study Group, 1991).

IV. CLINICAL TOXICITY OF INTERFERON-α

Adverse effects of interferon-α can be major obstacles to its clinical use. Particularly in early trials, the high dosage levels were associated with severe clinical toxicities in a typical pattern of early and late adverse effects (Table V). Several phase I studies and open studies with interferon-α-2c in patients suffering from advanced malignancies have identified a maximum tolerated dose (MTD) of 32.5×10^6 U/day i.m. Dose-limiting toxicity included fever, fatigue, loss of appetite, nausea, and chills. A few patients, in addition, exhibited severe neurotoxic symptoms. The acute toxicity of interferon-α-2c consists of constitutional symptoms that usually do not last longer than 1 or 2 weeks. The intensity was not only related to the dose but to the individual patient. The mechanism of fever induction is not clearly understood (increasing prostaglandin production in the hypothalamus?). Fatigue and

Table V. Typical Adverse Effects of Interferon-α

Early:	Fatigue[a]	Chills
	Fever[a]	Arthralgias
	Myalgias[a]	Headache
	Backache[a]	Nausea
	Anorexia[a]	Diarrhea
	Difficulty sleeping[a]	Abdominal cramps
	Impaired concentration[a]	
Late:	Bone marrow suppresion (mild)	
	Induction of neutralizing antibodies	
	Autoimmunity	
	Psychiatric disorders	
	Weight loss	
	Hair loss	

[a] May appear also after 2–6 weeks.

anorexia, often aggravated by nausea and eventually resulting in weight loss, were other dose-limiting toxicities of interferon-α-2c (Table VI).

Particularly when doses greater than 5×10^6 U of interferon-α-2c were administered, the nervous system became a target organ of chronic but reversible toxicity in a few patients. Symptoms included depression, confusion, and loss of concentration. As outlined by Bocci (1988), there is no clear dose-related neurotoxicity as a general rule. Age, on the other hand, appears as a predisposing factor for central nervous toxicity. Antecedent depressive states appear predisposing to depression. As discussed before, hematologic effects such as leukopenia appear frequently within hours of administration. However, they usually are not dose limiting, as thrombocytopenia rarely occurrs and is related to the dose and to the underlying disease.

Gastrointestinal toxicity included nausea, vomiting, and diarrhea. These symptoms were dose-dependent and adaptation occurred. Liver dysfunctions occurred in terms of elevated serum transaminases, usually more noticeable in patients who started therapy with elevated serum levels of transaminases.

The skin seemed to be a target of toxicity in a few patients receiving interferon-α-2c for longer periods. Thinning of the skin and mild hair loss have been reported; excessive growth of eyelashes occurred occasionally. Itching and rash due to interferon-α-2c were quite rare (Table VI). Other organ systems were not identified as typical targets of toxicity. Clinical toxicities were difficult to predict from the preclinical safety studies. Only fever, neurotoxicity, and the hematological adverse effects could be anticipated on the basis of the pharmacodynamic properties of interferon-α-2c.

Table VI. Adverse Events in Patients Treated with Interferon-α-2c for Indications other than Hairy Cell Leukemia[a]

Type of toxicity	Patients with symptom (%)[b]
Constitutional symptoms	
Fever	73
Fever, WHO grades III/IV	7
Pain	37
Appetite disturbance	27
Fatigue	24
Myalgia	18
Hypotension	16
Headache	16
Weakness	11
Chills	11
Arthralgia	7
Gastrointestinal symptoms	
Nausea, vomiting	8
Diarrhea	2
Neurological symptoms	
Depression	4
Confusion	2
Loss of concentration	1
Cutaneous symptoms	
Rash	6
Hair loss	5
Allergic reactions	2
Laboratory-related data	
Leukocytopenia	34
Lymphocytopenia	76
Granulocytopenia	34
Aspartate aminotransferase elevation	39
Alanine aminotransferase elevation	36
Blood urea nitrogen elevation	2

[a] Dosage: median, 3×10^6 U/day; range, $2–30 \times 10^6$ U/day; administered s.c./i.m.; 60% of the patients received concomitant therapy.
[b] $n = 392$.

As experience with the use of interferon-α-2c has grown, dosages have been lowered. In parallel, toxicities have decreased considerably. As shown in Table VII, a low dose of interferon-α-2c alfa-2c in patients with hairy cell leukemia reduced the frequency and severity of adverse events significantly without diminishing the efficacy of the long-term treatment.

Table VII. Adverse Events in Hairy Cell Leukemia Patients Treated with Interferon-α-2c

Type of toxicity	Dose	
	$1.6–5.0 \times 10^6$ U/day[a]	$0.5–1.6 \times 10^6$ U/day[b]
Fever, flu-like symptoms	27	0
Pain	13	1
Cytopenia	8	0
Gastrointestinal disorder	8	0
Hepatotoxicity	7	0
Fatigue	4	0
Hair loss	2	0
Neurological disorder	2	0
Hypotension	1	0
Impotency	1	0

[a] Values in table are numbers of patients with toxicity; $n = 63$.
[b] Values in table are numbers of patients with toxicity; $n = 46$.

The immunogenic potential (defined as the ability of epitopes to induce antibody formation) of the multiple recombinant and natural interferon-α preparations used in human therapy has become increasingly interesting in clinical research. In order to study the long-term immunogenicity of interferon-α-2c in cancer patients, ~2000 serum samples were screened for neutralizing antibodies to human interferon-α-2c based on their ability to inhibit the antiviral activity of the interferon (ANB assay). After long-term interferon-α-2c treatment, 346 patients were eligible for evaluation over a treatment period of 2–52 months. Most patients were treated longer than 6 months. Of the 346 patients, three (0.87%) exhibited measurable titers of neutralizing antibodies following therapy with interferon-α-2c; 163 patients suffered from non-Hodgkin's lymphomas, leukemias, and preleukemias. One patient with chronic myeloid leukemia experienced antibody induction under therapy, and 183 patients had solid tumors. Two of them reacted with antibody production. All titers were rather low (1:12, 1:8, and 1:64, respectively).

The clinical significance of antiinterferon-α antibodies is still under discussion. However, more and more reports indicate that relapses after successful interferon-α therapy coincide with the formation of neutralizing antibodies against interferon-α (Figlin *et al.,* 1988; Oberg and Alm, 1989; Steis *et al.,* 1988; von Wussow *et al.,* 1987, 1991; Itri *et al.,* 1989; Prümmer and Porzsolt, 1991). Because the ANB assay measures the inhibition of a pivotal pharmacodynamical function of interferon-α by specific antibodies, it is conceivable that the results of such studies may be important for the prediction of the long-term efficacy of treatment with a given interferon-α preparation. Data reported for other recombinant interferon-α trials (Figlin and Itri, 1988; Inglada *et al.,* 1987; Itri *et al.,* 1987; Jacobs and Kelsey, 1986; Spiegal *et al.,* 1989) differ markedly (Table VIII).

The rare antibody induction due to interferon-α-2c raises questions as to how the above-mentioned differences may be understood. Using X-ray crystallography, it has been shown that at least 15 amino acid residues may be implicated in each epitope. Functional approaches, such as studies of cross-reactive binding or studies with systematic replacements by other amino acids, have reduced this number to 1–3 residues and have shown that continuous epitopes are usually not longer than 7 residues (van Regenmortel, 1989). From theses studies one may conclude that replacements of single amino acids have significant influence on the immunogenicity of continuous and discontinuous epitopes.

Comparing recombinant interferon-α-2a, -2b, and -2c, the only available structural information is restricted to their linear scale of the 165 amino acid sequences. As shown in Table VIII, the differences occur at positions 23 and 34, with interferon-α-2c exhibiting arginines at both positions, interferon-α-2b exhibiting arginine at position 23 only, and interferon-α-2a exhibiting no arginines. In the study by Geysen *et al.* (1988) on the frequency of different amino acids in known immunogenic epitopes, one of the few clear-cut trends was that arginine was greatly underrepresented. This finding also explains the poor immunogenicity of histones—protein rich in this amno acid, even in their low immunogenic continuous epitopes (van Regenmortel, 1989; Getzoff *et al.,* 1988). As shown by Geysen *et al.* (1988), the propensity factors for the occurrence of each of the 20 common amino acids in sequential epitopes specific for critical residues is five times greater for histidine and lysine if compared with arginine.

The particularly low propensity for arginine to occur as a critical residue is also consistent with the finding that closely related proteins can be distinguished serologically, when they differ in an epitope that includes arginine in an unreactive protein and another amino acid residue in the reactive protein.

Table VIII. Structural Differences of Recombinant Interferon-α and Clinical Immunogenicity in Cancer Patients

Recombinant interferon	Amino acids in position		Induction rates of utralizing antibodies
	23	34	
IFN-α-2a	Lys	His	20–50%
IFN-α-2b	Arg	His	3–30%
IFN-α-2c	Arg	Arg	>1%

As discussed by Getzoff *et al.* (1988), the Oz locus of human IgG is a good example, in which Oz$^+$ equates to a lysine at position 193, and Oz$^-$, to arginine. It seems possible that the low clinical immunogenicity of interferon-α-2c is due to the relatively overrepresented arginine. It is important to note that both critical arginines of interferon-α-2c occur next to arginine residues conserved in all human interferon-α and -β species.

V. CLINICAL TOXICITY OF INTERFERON-γ

Patients with a variety of diseases, including advanced malignancies, viral infections, and psoriasis, were studied in clinical trials of the safety, efficacy, and tolerance of multiple-dose intramuscular administration of interferon-γ-1b. The percentage of patients experiencing clinical toxicities and laboratory abnormalities is shown in Table IX.

Clinical toxicity and laboratory abnormalities associated with interferon-γ-1b intramuscular administration are dose dependent and reversible on discontinuation of the drug. Sex of the patient does not appear to influence clinical toxicities, but laboratory abnormalities appear to increase with age. As is evident by comparing with clinical toxicities following subcutaneous administration, the frequency of constitutional symptoms related to intra-

Table IX. Adverse Events in Patients Treated with Interferon-γ-1b[a]

	Dose (μg/m^2)		
	50	100	>100
Clinical toxicity			
Myalgia	78	49	72
Fatigue	70	56	86
Headache	61	69	74
Fever	44	67	91
Chills	17	59	90
Nausea	13	31	53
Vomiting	13	13	34
Anorexia	4	18	52
Laboratory abnormalities			
Neutropenia	13	22	43
Thrombocytopenia	0	2	5
Serum glutamate oxalacetate transferase	0	3	21
Triglyceride elevation	0	18	36

[a] Administered i.m., n = 437. Values in the table are percentages of patients with adverse effects.

muscular administration of interferon-γ-1b is greater than when the same dose is administered subcutaneously.

More than 900 patients treated with interferon-γ-1b in single-agent clinical trials have been tested for the presence of antibody to interferon-γ by a sensitive radioimmunoprecipitation assay that detects neutralizing as well as nonneutralizing antibodies. All assays performed to date have been negative, with the exception of one patient, whose subsequent samples were negative (Jaffe *et al.,* 1987).

VI. CONCLUSION

Due to their species-restricted biological activities and their xenogenic immunogenicity, human interferons have posed a major problem to the preclinical prediction of safety and efficacy. Clinical experience yielded, particularly on high-dose treatment, some unforeseen toxicities, including isotypic immunogenicity of human interferon-α. In human therapy, a clear dose–response relationship is still lacking. Nevertheless, the continuous reduction of the interferon doses in clinical trials has led to tremendous reduction in the frequency and severity of adverse effects without losing efficacy.

References

Bocci, V. (1988). *J. Biol. Regul. Homeostatic Agents* **2**, 107–118.

Buchmeier, N. A., and Schreiber, R. D. (1985). *Proc. Natl. Acad. Sci. U.S.A.* **82**, 7404–7408.

Chen, B. D.-M., and Najor, F. (1987). *Cell. Immunol.* **106**, 343.

Curnutte, J. D., Berkow, R. L., Roberts, R. L., Shurin, S. B., and Scott, P. J. (1988). *Blood* **81**, 606–610.

DePaoli, A., Johnson, D. O., and Noll, W. W. (1973). *J. Am. Med. Assoc.* **163**, 624.

Dworkin-Rastl, E., Dworkin, M. B., and Swetly, P. (1982). *J. Interferon Res.* **2**, 575–585.

Dworkin-Rastl, E., Swetly, P., and Dworkin, M. B. (1983). *Gene* **20**, 237–248.

Fattorossi, A., Dolei, A., Pizollo, J. G., Cafolla, A., Mandelli, F., and Dianzani, F. (1987). *J. Biol. Regul. Homeostatic Agents* **1**, 87–92.

Figlin, R. M., and Itri, L. M. (1988). *Semin. Hematol.* **25**(3), 9–15.

Figlin, R. A., deKernion, J. B., Mukamel, E., Palleroni, A. V., Itri, L. M., and Sarna, G. P. (1988). *J. Clin. Oncol.* **6**, 1604–1610.

Genot, E., Billard, C., Sigaux, F., Mathiot, C., Degos, L., Falcoff, E., and Kolb, J. P. (1987). *Leukemia* **1**, 590–596.

Getzoff, E. D., Tainer, J. A., Lerner, R. A., and Geysen, H. M. (1988). *Adv. Immunol.* **43**, 1–89.

Geysen, H. M., Mason, T. J., and Rodda, S. J. (1988). *J. Mol. Recognition* **1**, 32–41.

Goeddel, D. V., Leung, D. W., Dull, T. J., Gross, M., Lawn, R. M., McCandless, R., Seeburg, P. H., Ulrich, A., Yelverton, E., and Gray, P. W. (1981) *Nature (London)* **290**, 20.

Inglada, L., Porres, J. C., LaBanda, F., Mora, I., and Carreno, V. (1987). *Lancet ii,* 1521.

International Chronic Granulomatous Disease Cooperative Study Group (1991). *N. Engl. J. Med.* **324**, 509–516.

Isaacs, A., and Lindenmann, J. (1957). *Proc. R. Soc. London, Ser. B* **147**, 258–267.

Itri, L. M., Campion, M., Denning, R. A., Palleroni, A. V., Guttermann, J. U., Groopman, J. E., and Trown, P. W. (1987). *Cancer* (Philadelphia) **59**, 668–674.

Itri, L. M., Sherman, M. I., Palleroni, A. V., Evans, L. M., Tran, L. L., Campion, M., and Chizzonite, R. (1989). *J. Interferon Res.* **9**, 9–16.

Jacobs, S. L., and Kelsey, D. K. (1986). *N. Engl. J. Med.* **315**, 1418.

Jaffe, H. S., and Sherwin, S. A. (1986). *In* "Interferons as Cell Growth Inhibitors and Antitumor Factors" (R. M. Friedman, T. Merigan, and T. Sreevalsan, eds.), pp. 509–522. Alan R. Liss, New York.

Jaffe, H. S., Chen, A. B., Kramer, S., and Sherwin S. A. (1987). *J. Biol. Response Modif.* **6**, 576–580.

Kiderlen, A. F., Kaufmann, S. H. E., and Lohmann-Matthes, M. L. (1984). *Eur. J. Immunol.* **14**, 964–967, 1984.

McCabe, R. E., Luft, B. J., and Remington, J. S. (1984). *J. Infect. Dis.* **150**, 961–962.

Murray, H. W., Rubin, B. Y., and Rothermel, C. D. (1983). *J. Clin. Invest.* **72**, 1506–1510.

Nathan, C. F., Murray, H. W., Wiebe, M. E., and Rubin, B. Y. (1983). *J. Exp. Med.* **158**, 670–689.

Nerl, C., Lander, T., Thaller, J. B., Neumann, K., Zachoval, R., and Kaboth, W. (1989). *J. Interferon Res.* **9**, 138. (Abstr.)

Neuman, H. A., and Fauser, A. A. (1982). *Exp. Hematol.* **10**, 587–590.

Oberg, K. (1988). *J. Interferon Res.* **8**, 22. (Abstr.)

Oberg, K., and Alm, G. (1989). *J. Interferon Res.* **9**, 45–49.

Oladipupo-Williams, C. K., Svet-Moldavskaya, I., and Bilchek, J. (1981). *Oncology* **38**, 356–360.

Paganelli, K. A., Evan, S. S., Han, T., and Ozer, T. (1986). *Blood* **67**, 937–942.

Prümmer, O., and Porzsolt, F. (1991). *Eur. Interferon Workshop, 6th, Hannover* Abstr., p. 20.

Sigaux, F., Castaigne, S., Lehn, P., Dupuy, P., Billard, C., Gluckman, J. C., Boiron, M., Falcoff, E., Flandrin, G., and Degos, L. (1987). *Int. J. Cancer* **1**, 2–8.

Spiegel, R. J., Jacobs, S. L., and Treuhaft, M. W. (1989). *J. Interferon Res.* (*Suppl. 1*) **9**, S14–17.

Steis, R. G., Smith, J. W., II, Urba, W., Clark, J. W., Itri, L. M., Evans, L. M., Schoenberger, C., and Longo, D. L. (1988). *N. Engl. J. Med.* **318**, 1409–1413.

Strander, H. (1986). *Adv. Cancer Res.* **47**, 66–68.

Streuli, M., Nagata, S. and Weissmann, C. (1980). *Science* **209**, 1343–1347.

Tanaka, T., and Craig, A. W. (1970). *Eur. J. Cancer* **6**, 329.

Trent, J. M., Olsson, S., and Lawn, R. M. (1982). *Proc. Natl. Acad. Sci. U.S.A.* **79**, 7809–7813.

van Regenmortel, M. H. V. (1989). *Immunol. Today* **10**, 266–272.

Verma, D. S., Spitzer, G., and Gutterman, J. U. (1978). *Blood* **54**, 1423–1427.

von Wussow, P., Freund, M., Block, B., Poliwoda, H., and Deicher, H. (1987). *Lancet* (Sept. 12), 635–636.

von Wussow, P., Pralle, H., Jakschies, D., and Deicher, H. (1991). *Eur. Interferon Workshop, 6th, Hannover* Abstr., p. 23.

Clinical Experience with *Escherichia coli* rHuGM-CSF

Angelika C. Stern and Thomas C. Jones
Clinical Research
Sandoz Pharma Ltd.
CH-4002 Basel, Switzerland

I. INTRODUCTION

Colony-stimulating factors (CSFs) are low-molecular-weight glycoproteins
that are necessary for the survival, proliferation, and differentiation of hematopoietic progenitors (Peters, 1991). In the natural state these factors
are glycosylated, but the use of bacterially synthesized (*Escherichia coli*-
derived) human recombinant granulocyte–macrophage CSF (rHuGM-CSF)
in clinical trials showed that glycosylation does not appear to be essential
for biological activity. This article will review the studies done with *E.
coli*-derived rHuGM-CSF, which present evidence of reversal of neu-
tropenic states, and determine whether this reversal leads, as predicted, to
clinically relevant patient benefits.

GM-CSF is not meant to cure a specific disease, but to act as adjunct
therapy in a number of conditions that are associated with bone marrow
failure. Data on the effects of GM-CSF in preventing or treating myeloid
hypoplasia after cytotoxic chemotherapy in cancer, on myeloid recovery
after bone marrow transplantation, and as an adjunct to therapy in diseases

of dysmyelopoiesis [myelodysplastic syndrome (MDS), aplastic anemia (AA), and acquired immune deficiency syndrome (AIDS)] will be presented.

II. EFFICACY OF GM-CSF IN PREVENTION AND TREATMENT OF MYELOID HYPOPLASIA AFTER CHEMOTHERAPY FOR CANCER

Chemotherapy of cancer has been shown to be valuable in contributing to long-term survival and even cure in a number of human malignancies (DeVita, 1989). However, a major side effect of these drugs is myelotoxicity (Pizzo, 1984), which causes two major clinical problems; first, the occurrence of infection during the myelosuppressive period, leading to prolonged hospitalization, excessive antibiotic use, and patient morbidity and mortality (Schimpff, 1990; DeVita, 1989); second, the inability to maintain the dose of chemotherapy known to be effective in inducing prolonged remission or cure of the cancer. GM-CSF has therefore been evaluaed in this setting to determine whether it can prevent or reverse the myelosuppression and if it can then reduce the associated infections and allow adherence to the cancer chemotherapy schedule.

A. Prevention of Neutropenia after Cancer Chemotherapy

One study, a multicenter study of patients with small cell lung cancer (SCCL), compared two different dose groups (10 and 20 μg/kg daily, given as a single dose, subcutaneously) with an untreated observation group (Schiller *et al.,* 1990). The study showed that the use of GM-CSF led to significantly shorter periods of neutropenia and the depth of the nadir was less profound in patients receiving GM-CSF. These results are consistent with the results seen in other studies. In addition, there was evidence of better delivery of full cytotoxic chemotherapy. This, however, resulted in increased evidence of megakaryocytic toxicity in cycles 3–6. The infection rate in all groups was relatively low, therefore, no effect on the occurrence of infection was identified. It was shown that the 10-μg/kg daily dose was as effective as the 20-μg/kg dose and slightly better tolerated. Two additional studies have been completed and are now being analyzed (one in germ cell carcinoma, one in non-Hodgkin's lymphoma) and show reduction of infection complications during chemotherapy and better adherence to the chemotherapy protocols.

A dose-finding study in non-Hodgkin's lymphoma contributed to defining the dose range of GM-CSF (5.5–11 μg/kg) for chemotherapy protocols with moderate myelotoxicity (less than seen in the SCCL study) and also showed that once-daily subcutaneous dosing for 5 days yielded the same result as a twice-daily regimen. This supports the recommendation of a dose range from 5 to 10 μg/kg, depending on the underlying disease and degree of chemotherapy (Hovgaard and Nissen, 1991). This study also contributed to the understanding that there is no difference in glycosylated mammalian-derived rHuGM-CSF and *E. coli*-derived rHuGM-CSF with respect to clinical efficacy and safety.

B. Treatment of Established Neutropenia after Cancer Chemotherapy

The efficacy of GM-CSF in the treatment of established neutropenia primarily occurring after cancer chemotherapy was studied. A study perfomed by Gerhartz *et al.* (1989,1991) confirmed that GM-CSF reverses the neutropenia within 1–3 days, which is clearly shorter than the 10 days required in the placebo arm of the study. This study also showed that doses of 5.5–11 μg/kg once daily is the appropriate dose, as 1.4 and 2.8 μg/kg did not lead to a significant benefit. This study showed also that glycosylated rHuGM-CSF has the same efficacy and safety as nonglycosylated rHuGM-CSF and demonstrated a similar effect in intravenous and subcutaneous aplication. Another study showed that there is no evidence of intolerance of GM-CSF in the presence of bacterial sepsis (Biesma *et al.*, 1990).

An open study using a compassionate-need protocol evaluated the role of GM-CSF in patients with prolonged neutropenia after cancer chemotherapy or bone marrow engraftment failure. Over 80% of the patients showed reversal of their neutropenia within 2–4 days when they were treated with 400 μg daily for 3–28 days (Helg *et al.*, 1990).

III. EFFICACY OF GM-CSF IN ASSOCIATION WITH BONE MARROW TRANSPLANTATION

Though the administration of large doses of chemotherapy agents potentially increases the anticancer response, it also normally increases the toxicity, particularly the myelotoxicity. One possibility to overcome this myelotoxicity after very high doses of chemotherapy with or without radiation is the reinfusion of previously harvested and stored autologous bone marrow (ABM) (Herzig, 1981; Souhami and Peters, 1986; Phillips *et al.*, 1984). In this setting, all patients have granulocyte counts $<500/\mu$l and are therefore at serious risk for life-threatening infection. Any measure encouraging hematopoiesis and a quick increase in granulocyte count $\geq500/\mu$l would be of direct benefit for the patients.

A total of 231 patients with various tumors and after various preparative regimens were enrolled at 20 centers into a double-blind, placebo-controlled study of the use of GM-CSF after autologous bone marrow transplantation. GM-CSF was administered until the patient reached a granulocyte count of over $1000/\mu l$ for three consecutive days, or, if this did not occur, for a period of not more than 30 days. All patients were assessed for efficacy of treatment. One center harvested peripheral blood stem cells in addition to bone marrow in an effort to increase the number of transplanted cells. These patients were evaluated separately.

The median time after transplantation until the recovery of granulocyte counts greater than $500/\mu l$ was determined. Overall, this was significantly shorter in the GM-CSF-treated group as compared with the placebo group. The percentage of patients with myeloid cell increases above $500 /\mu l$ on day 19 was also significantly higher in the GM-CSF treatment group. In some subgroups of patients these differences were particularly notable (Visani *et al.,* 1991).

The effects of earlier recovery times on other clinical parameters were examined. GM-CSF produced a trend toward improved clinical outcome in the analyses, but these results wee not statistically significant in all cases. Biochemical parameters of organ toxicity significantly improved (decreased bilirubin) and key features such as days in isolation and days in intensive care unit and hospital days decreased significantly. These parameters are viewed as the primary indicators of patient well-being. Antibiotic usage did not show a difference, but this may reflect current empiric antibiotic protocols because, in the analysis of one center, a decrease in antibiotic use was a major factor in decreased costs (Bennett *et al.,* 1990). These benefits are similar to those recently reported by Nemunaitis *et al.* (1991) in which decreased hospitalization from 33 days to 28 days was the major benefit. Infections did not occur as frequently in patients receiving GM-CSF but the differences were not statistically significant.

IV. EFFICACY OF GM-CSF IN DISEASES CHARACTERIZED BY DYSMYELOPOIESIS

Myelodysplastic syndrome (MDS) is a diverse group of disorders. These syndromes range from chronic, mild anemias with little propensity to evolve to acute leukemia (estimated at 7%), to disorders in which there are profound abnormalities in the production of all blood elements (i.e., severe anemia, leukopenia, and/or thrombocytopenia). Most patients present with pancytopenia, usually involving two or more cell lines (platelets, erythrocytes, leukocytes) without an obvious explanation for bone marrow failure. Cytogenetic abnormalities occur in 20–60% of patients. Morphological characteristics of bone marrow in MDS patients include disorders in the formation of erythrocytic, granulocytic, and megakaryocytic cell lineages; increases in blast cell number and abnormal bone marrow histology are common (Bennett, 1986).

The goals for the use of a molecule such as rHuGM-CSF would be to reduce morbidity from infection in milder forms of the disease, and to increase responsiveness to chemotherapy in those forms likely to progress to leukemia. The dangers of rHuGM-CSF if used inappropriately would be the potential conversion of mild disease forms to leukemic progressive forms. This issue has been addressed in both the design and the evaluation of all the clinical trials.

Aplastic Anemia (AA) is a stem cell disorder characterized by fatty replacement of hematopoietic tissue and pancytopenia. In contrast to MDS, cytogenetic abnormalities are rare. The clinical presentation of aplastic anemia is similar to MDS in that it represents yet another bone marrow failure state. The bone marrow is usually aplastic or hypocellular. Patients incur anemia, leukopenia, or thrombocytopenia; their disease course is thus characterized by recurrent infections and bleeding (Camitta *et al.*, 1982). A major distinction from MDS is the higher degree of bone marrow damage in aplastic anemia, occasionally with complete absence of bone marrow cells. This difference predicts that responses to a molecule such as rHuGM-CSF, which induces proliferation of existing cells at a rate approximately three times faster than under normal hematopoiesis, will not be so dramatic in aplastic anemia, and indeed some patients with severe AA will not be expected to respond at all.

The study in MDS is a randomized parallel group study comparing the use of GM-CSF to standard management of an observation group of patients with well-characterized MDS according to the French–American–British (FAB) classification (Schuster *et al.*, 1990). The study involved 27 investigators who enrolled 133 patients with MDS, of which 122 patients could be evaluated for efficacy. Data are available on patients observed for up to 12 weeks, although some patients were subsequently followed during long-term treatment with GM-CSF or were observed without long-term treatment. A dose of 3 μg/kg daily by single subcutaneous injection was used in the majority of patients. Patients at high risk for leukemia (i.e., more than 15% blasts in the bone marrow) were not included.

The major effect of GM-CSF was a dramatic increase to normal levels of the granulocyte count. The question of clinical benefit resulting from the increase of granulocytes was addressed by evaluating the total number of infections and the number of serious infections. The increase in granulocyte count was accompanied by a statistically significant decrease ($p = 0.03$) in the number of serious infections. Ten of the 61 patients in the GM-CSF group versus 19 of 61 patients in the observation group had serious infections. The adverse events are reported in Section V of this report; however, of particular note is that leukemic conversions, a part of the natural history of MDS, occurred in four patients after receiving GM-CSF (6%) and in three patients in the observation group. (5%). This was consistent with the natural history of this disease. The study therefore shows both an increase in circulating white blood cells and a decrease in serious infections without contributing to the major potential problem of increased conversion of MDS patients to leukemia. The problems of thrombocytopenia or anemia are not solved by this molecule; however, they are not exacerbated.

The multicenter study also enrolled patients with aplastic anemia; 41 patients were assessed. Patients had to have moderately severe aplastic anemia that had failed to respond to previous therapy; however, marrow fibrosis was an exclusion criteria. Severe neutropenia (below 400 granulocytes/μl) was demonstrated. During 1–3 months of treatment, a significant increase in granulocyte numbers was observed. In this study control of infections was significantly affected by use of GM-CSF. Infections were common in both patient groups but major infections occurred at a different frequency in the two groups. Of the GM-CSF group, 30% had major infections (defined in the protocol as requiring hospitalization and intravenous antibiotics); however, only one patient had documented infection. No bacteremia, fungemia, or pneumonias were recorded during the 3-month period. In contrast, 56% of the patients in the observation group had major infections; seven patients were given active drug treatment because of the infection. These infections included aspergillus pneumonia, gram-positive and gram-negative bacteremia, cellulitis, *Klebsiella* pneumonia, and bacterial sinusitis.

Neutropenia, either spontaneous or treatment induced, is an important factor limiting treatment options for patients with acquired immune deficiency syndrome. A relatively small proportion of patients with AIDS present with life-threatening neutropenia. However, a far larger proportion appears to be particularly susceptible to neutropenia induced by antiviral agents such as zidovudine (AZT) or ganciclovir (DHPG). One study used GM-CSF in combination with zidovudine plus interferon-α (Davey *et al.,* 1991). Low-dose GM-CSF (less than 1 μg/kg daily) ameliorated the neutropenia associated with zidovudine and interferon-α therapy without adversly affecting the antiviral properties of the combination. The projected benefit in treatment of AIDS patients with GM-CSF is likely to be in allowing the use of full doses of concomitant antiviral or antitumor medications.

V. TOLERABILITY

The following mild to moderate adverse events are to be expected but are not usually treatment limiting: fever, myalgias, malaise, local reaction at injection site, and rash (Schiller *et al.,* 1990; Gerhartz *et al.,* 1989,1991; Hovgaard and Nissen, 1991; Helg *et al.,* 1990; Visani *et al.,* 1991; Schuster *et al.,* 1990; Davey *et al.,* 1991; Lieschke *et al.,* 1989,1990). Regarding the occurrence of side effects in the placebo-treated patients, each of these may be confused with the signs and symptoms of the underlying illness. At appropriate doses for each indication, these should be only mild or moderate in severity and should not occur in more than 20–30% of patients. They should be less of a problem than the risk of infection due to continual neutropenia or delayed bone marrow engraftment.

Serious reactions should be rare when proper doses are used (i.e., 5–10 μg/kg daily). They include inflammation of the pleura, pericardium, and endothelium. Continuous attention to their occurrence will be required. As recorded in these studies, unusual events such as allergic reactions, first-dose dyspnea, and unexplained leukocytosis will occasionally occur in spite of appropriate dosing. Careful monitoring must be a hallmark of the use of such a potent molecule.

Review of the tolerability data confirms that, with the higher doses of GM-CSF (above 10 μg/kg), an increase in mild to moderate adverse events can be expected, and more serious adverse events of pericarditis, hypotension, and respiratory distress can be observed. A warning against the tendency to increase doses in unresponding patients is included in the information concerning the use of GM-CSF. In special patient populations potential dangers need to be emphasized; in MDS there is a need to pay special attention to patients with >20% blasts in the bone marrow, thrombocytopenia, and bleeding; in lung cancer, pericarditis and respiratory distress, hypoxia, and hypotension with the first dose; in BMT, capillary leak syndrome and pericarditis; and in AIDS, thrombocytopenia and increased fatigue. When attention to dose and problems in special populations are considered, the drug has been shown to be safe and well tolerated with a high patient benefit-to-risk ratio. Long-term use has been evaluated in some patients and appears safe but needs further evaluation.

VI. SUMMARY AND CONCLUSION

The use of rHuGM-CSF has resulted in patient benefit as shown by reduced infections (MDS and AA), reduced days in intensive care (ABM transplant), better adherence to cancer chemotherapy protocols, and the ability to use full doses of antiviral drugs in AIDS and cytomegalovirus retinitis. The adverse reactions are significant when high doses are used, therefore high doses should be avoided (there is a plateau in the dose-effective biological responses). At recommended doses, GM-CSF is well tolerated and is a valuable adjunctive therapy in the management of patients with conditions of dysmyelopoiesis and myeloid hypoplasia associated with myelotoxic therapy, or after bone marrow transplantation.

References

Bennett, C. L., Greenberg, P., Gulati, S. C., Advani, R., and Bonnem, E. (1990). *Blood* **76**, Suppl. 1, 518A.

Bennett, J. M. (1986). *Clin. Haematol.* **15**, 909.

Biesma, B., DeVries, E. G. E., Willemse, P. H. B., Sluiter, W. J., Postmus, P. E., Limburg, P. C., Stern, A. C., and Vellenga, E. (1990). *Eur. J. Cancer* **26**, 932.

Camitta, B. M., Storb, R., and Thomas, E. D. (1982). *N. Engl. J. Med.* **306**, 645.

Davey, R. T., Davey, V. J., Metcalf, J. A., Zurlo, J. J., Kovacs, J. A., Falloon, J., Polis, M. A., Zunich, K. M., Masur, H., and Lane, H. C. (1991). *J. Infect. Dis.* **164**, 43.

DeVita, V. T. (1989). *In* "Cancer: Principles and Practice of Oncology" (V. T. DeVita, S. Hellmann, and S. A. Rosenberg, eds.), pp. 276–300. Lippincott, Philadelphia.

Gerhartz, H. H., Stern, A. C., Schmetzer, H., Wolf-Hornung, B., and Wilmanns, W. (1989). *Mol. Biother.* **1**, Suppl. 1, 22. (Abstr.)

Gerhartz, H. H., Stern, A. C., Wolf-Hornung, B., Kazempour, M., Schmetzer, H., Beykirch, M., Gugerli, U., and Wilmanns, W. (1991). *In* "Breakthrough in Cytokine Therapy: An Overview of GM–CSF" (J. H. Scarffe, ed.), R. Soc. Med. Serv. Int. Congr. Symp. Ser., No. 170, pp. 79–93. R. Soc. Med. Serv., London.

Helg, C., Froidevaux, P., Laurencet, F., Jeannet, M., and Chapuis, B. (1990). *Schweiz. Med. Wochenschr.* **120**, Suppl. 32/1, 408.

Herzig, G. P. (1981). *Prog. Hematol.* **12**, 1.

Hovgaard, D., and Nissen, N. I. (1991). *In* "Breakthrough in Cytokine Therapy: An Overview of GM–CSF" (J. H. Scarffe, ed.), Royal Soc. Med. Serv. Int. Congr. Symp. Ser., No. 170, pp. 71–78. Royal Soc. Med. Serv., London.

Lieschke, G. J., Cebon, J., and Morstyn, G. (1989). *Blood* **74**, 2634.

Lieschke, G. J., Maher, D., O'Connor, M., Green, M., Sheridan, W., Rallings, M., Bonnem, E., Burgess, A. W., McGrath, K., Fox, R. M., and Morstyn, G. (1990). *Cancer Res.* **50**, 614.

Nemunaitis, J., Rabinowe, S. N., Singer, J. W., Bierman, P. J., Vose, J. M., Freedman, A. S., Onetto, N., Gillis, S., Oette, D., Gold, M., Buckner, C. D., Hansen, J. A., Ritz, J., Appelbaum, F. R., Armitage, J. O., and Nadler, L. M. (1991). *N. Engl. J. Med.* **324**, 1773.

Peters, W. P. (1991). *Semin. Hematol.* **28**(2), Suppl. 2, 1.

Phillips, G. L., Herzig, R. H., and Lazarus, H. M. (1984). *N. Engl. J. Med.* **310**, 1557.

Pizzo, P. A. (1984). *Cancer (Philadelphia)* **54**, 2649.

Schiller, J. H., Storer, B., Oken, M. M., Saphner, T., Blank, J., Kohler, P., Weresch, J., Stone, W., O'Connel, K., and Aughey, J. (1990). *Proc. ASCO* **9**, 943. (Abstr.)

Schimpff, S. C. (1990). *In* "Principles and Practice of Infectious Diseases" (G. L. Mandell, ed.), pp. 2258–2264. Churchill-Livingstone, New York.

Schuster, M. W., Thompson, J. A., Larson, R., Allen, S. L., O'Laughlin, R., Israel, R., and Fefer, A. (1990). *Proc. ASCO* **9**, 793. (Abstr.)

Souhami, R., and Peters, W. (1986). *Clin. Haematol.* **15**, 219.

Visani, G., Gamberi, B., Greenberg, P., Advani, R., Gulati, S., Champlin, R., Hoglund, M., Karanes, C., Williams, S., Keating, A., Gyger, M., Pouillart, P., Gorin, N. C., Jacobson, R., Rybka, W., Syman, M., Poynton, C. H., Bjorkstrand, B., Santini, G., Tura, S., Powles, R. L., Stryckmans, P. A., Biggs, J., and Bonnem, E. (1991). *Bone Marrow Transplant.* **7**, Suppl 2, 81.

Index

Contents of Recent Volumes

ISBN 0-12-364935-8